Nurse's Diagnosis
A Nurse Coloring Book
Of Snarky, Sweary Nurse Humor

By Peaceful Mind Adult Coloring Books

Copyright © 2017

All rights reserved. No part of this publication may be reproduced, distributed, or transmitted in any form or by any means, including photocopying, recording, or other electronic or mechanical methods, without the prior written permission of the publisher

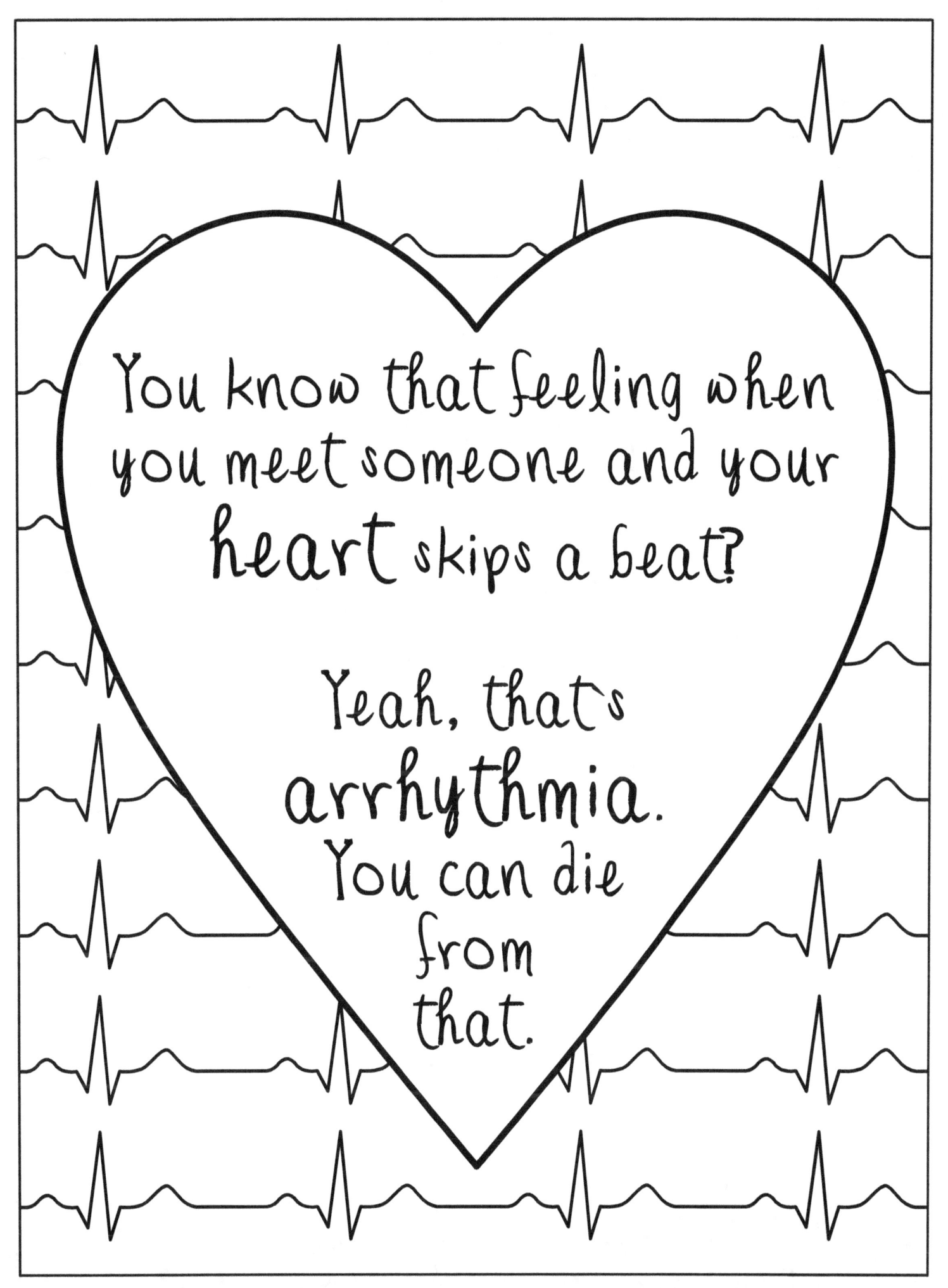

YES, I CHARTED THAT I CHARTED WHAT I PREVIOUSLY CHARTED. WAIT, HOLD ON. I HAVE TO CHART THAT I TOLD YOU ABOUT MY CHARTING.

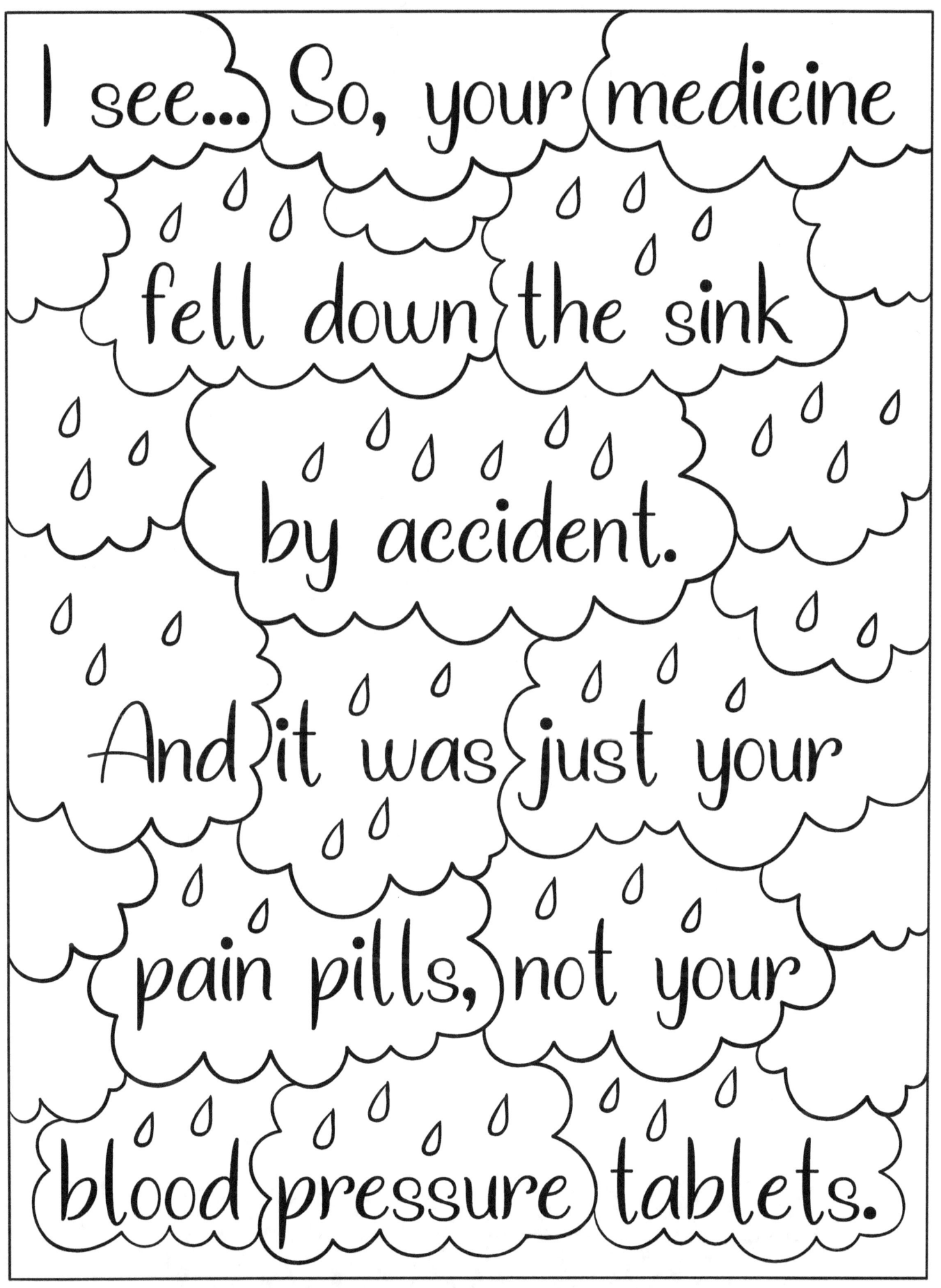

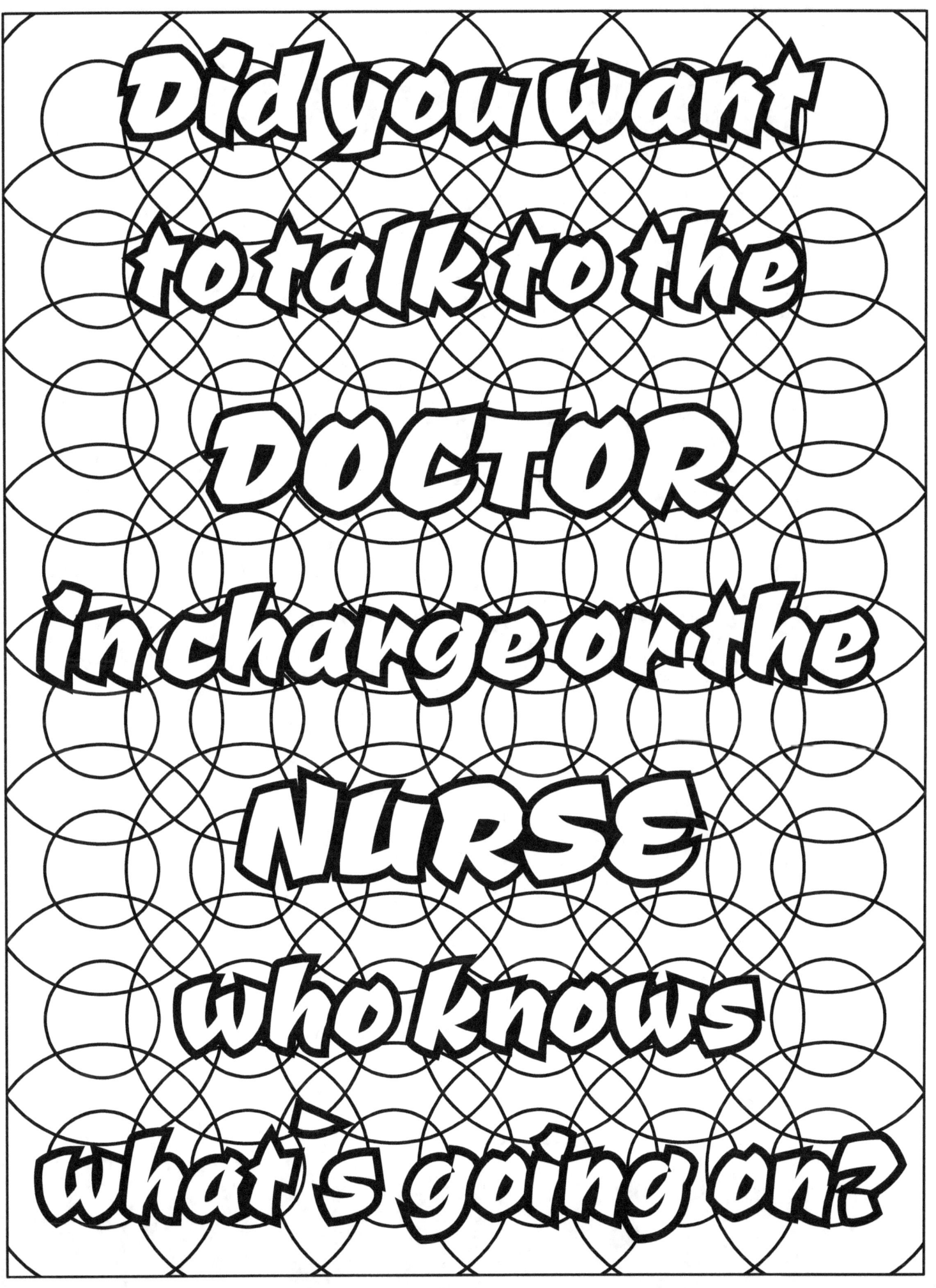

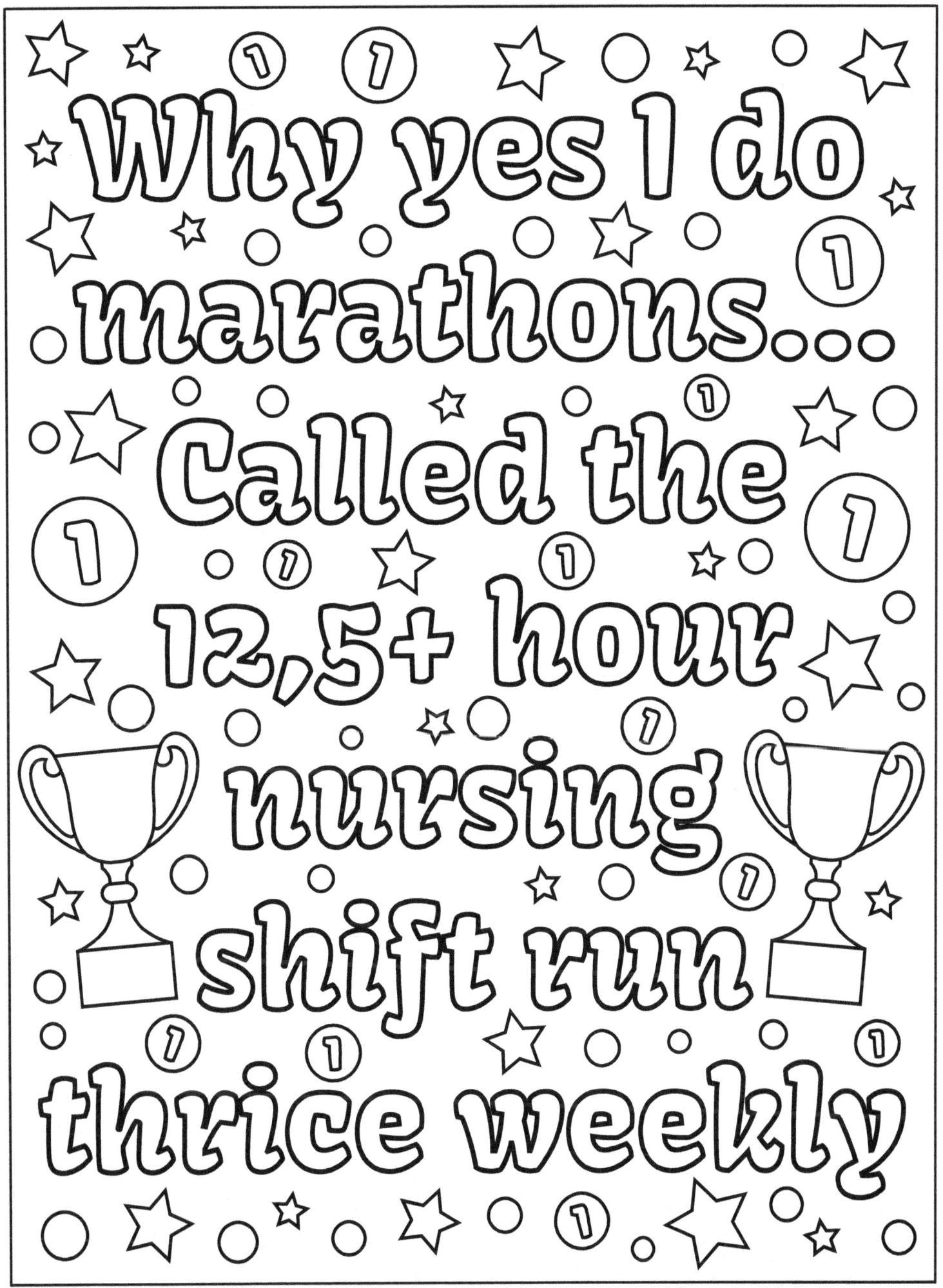

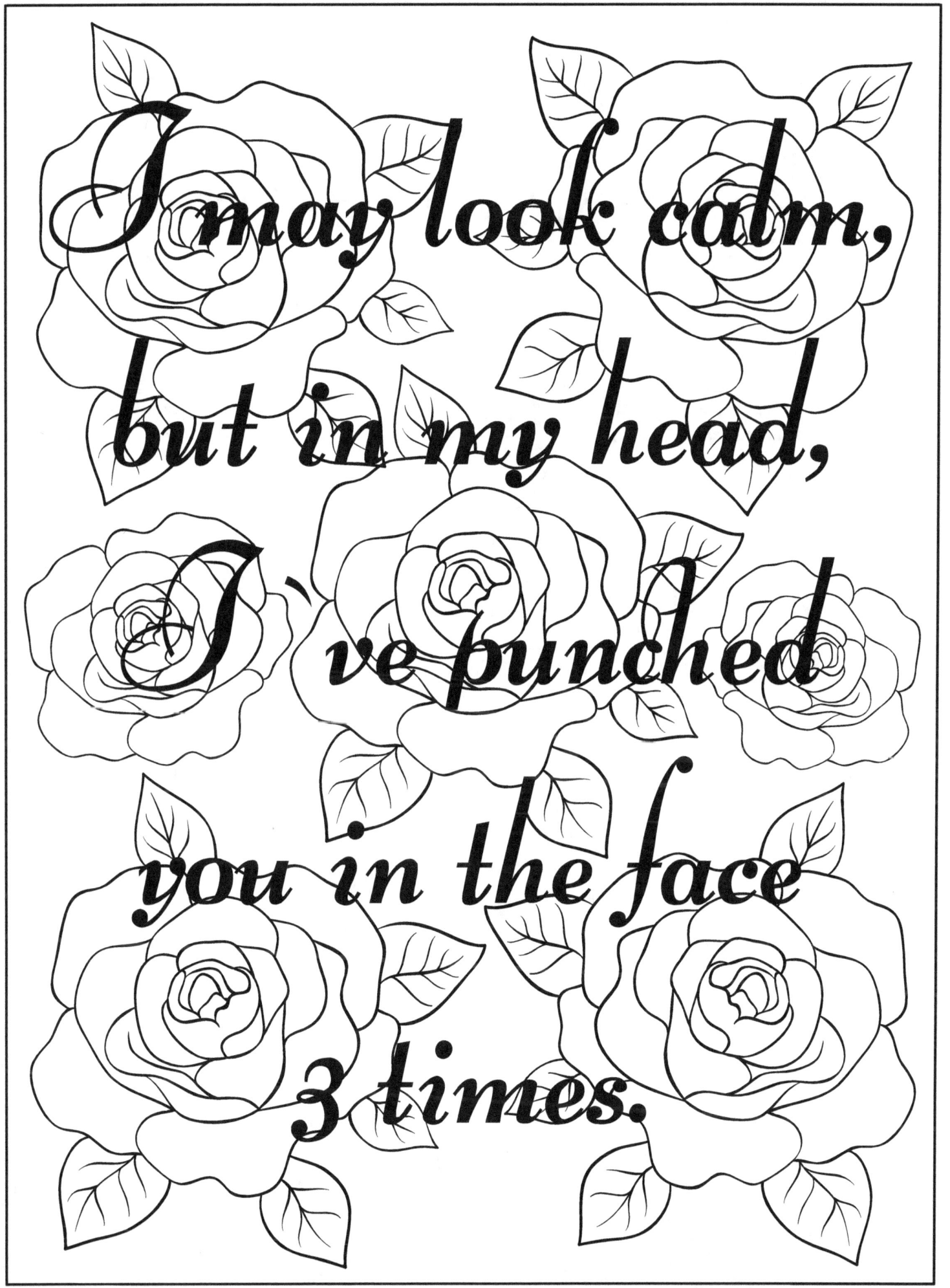

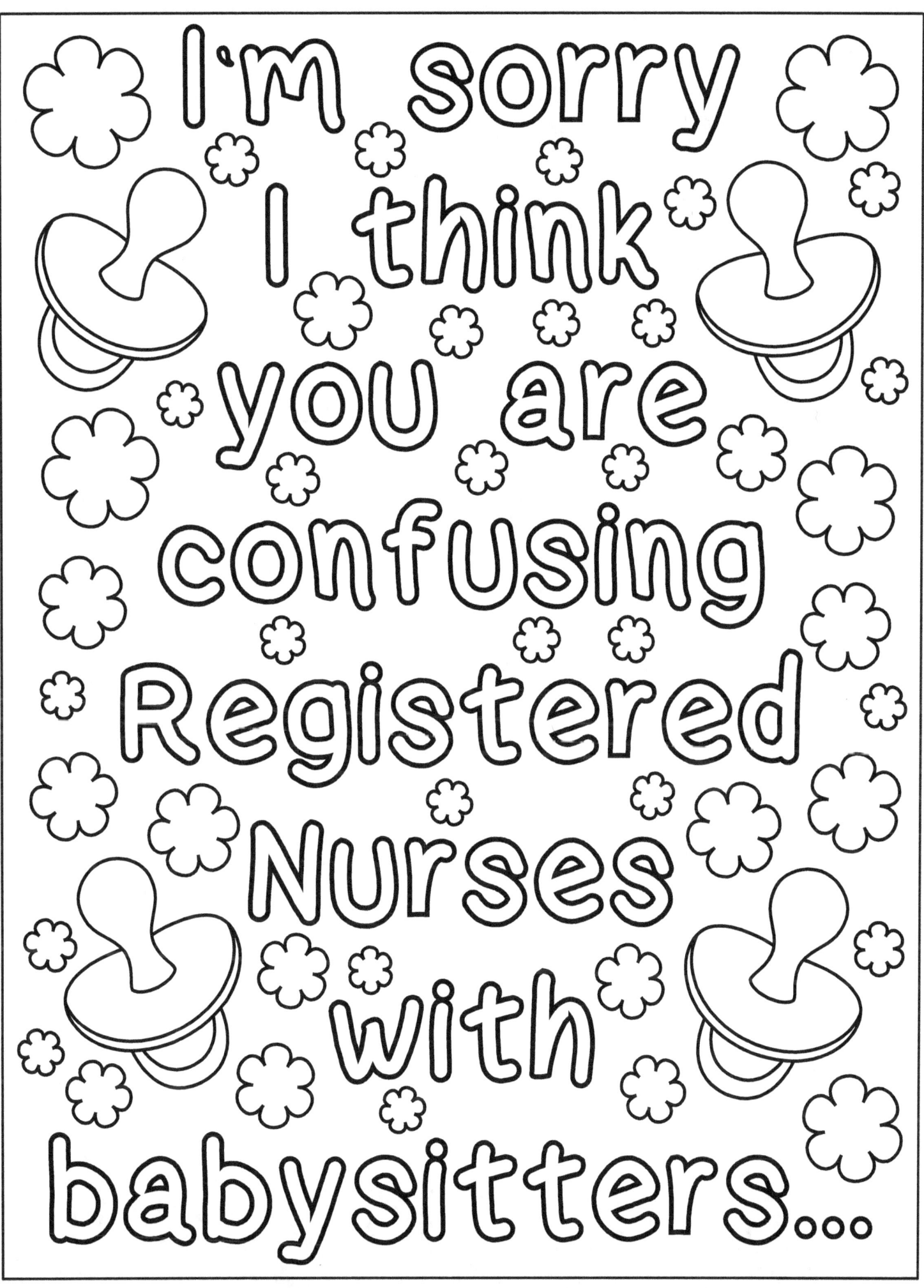

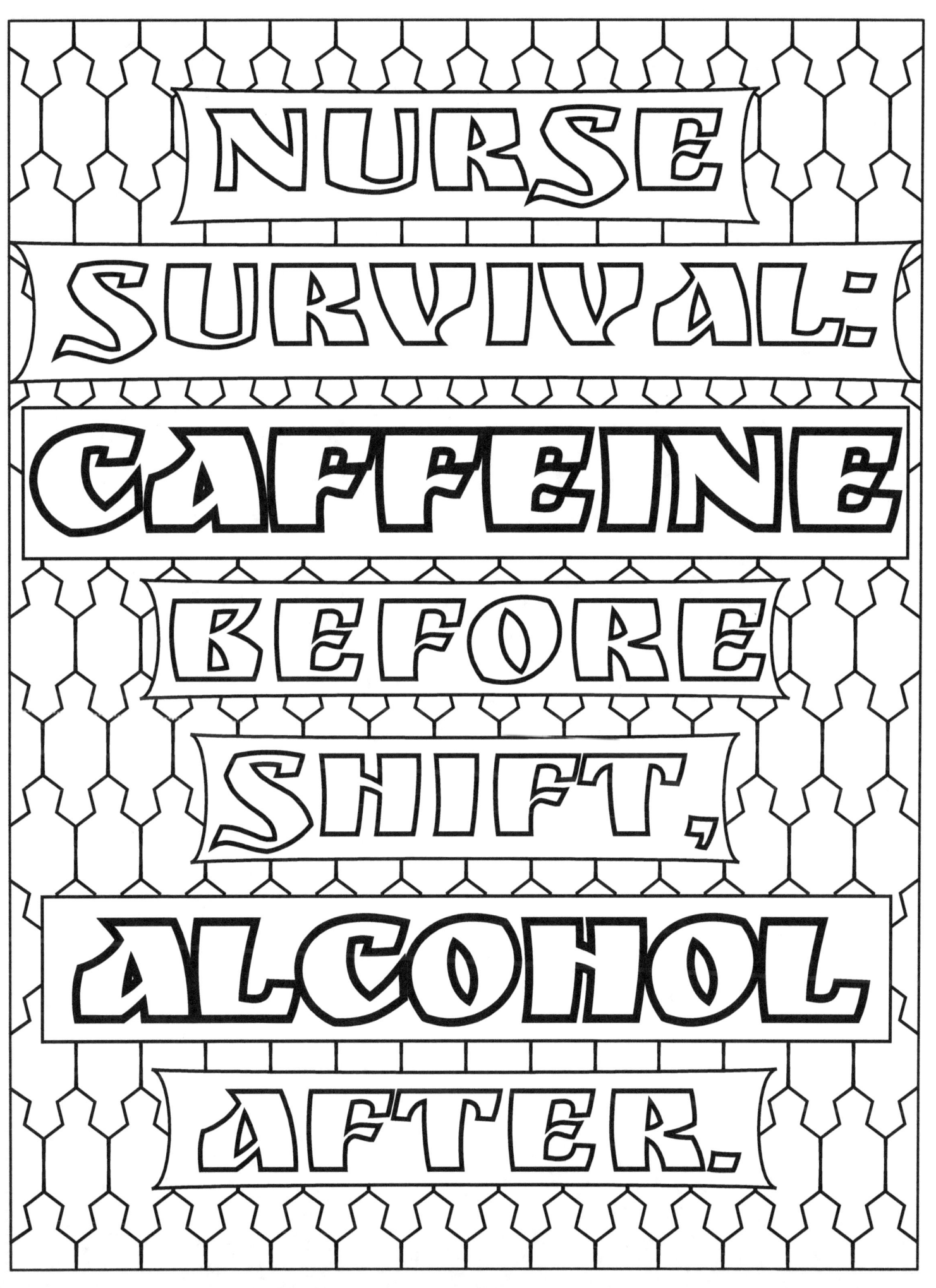

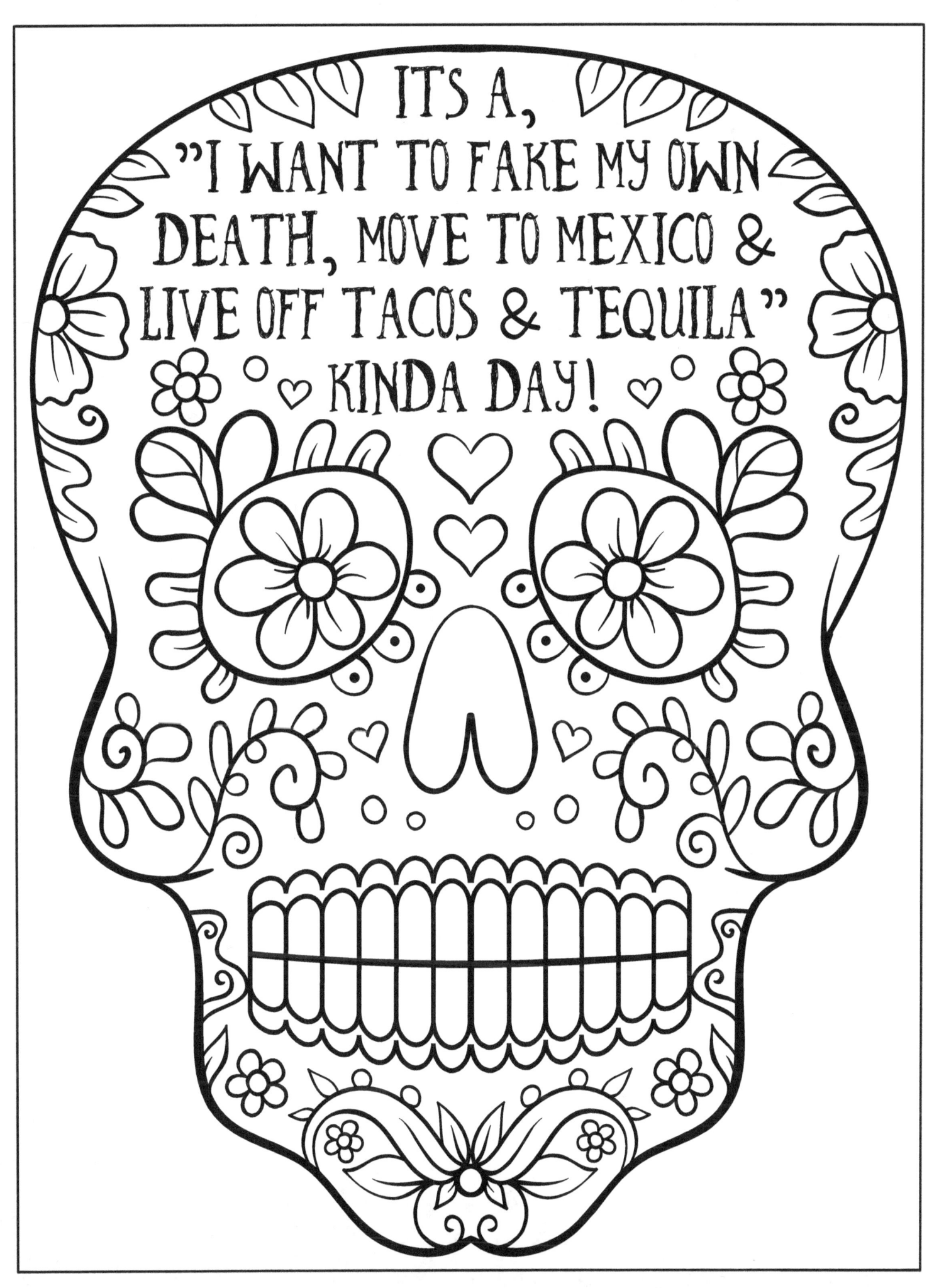

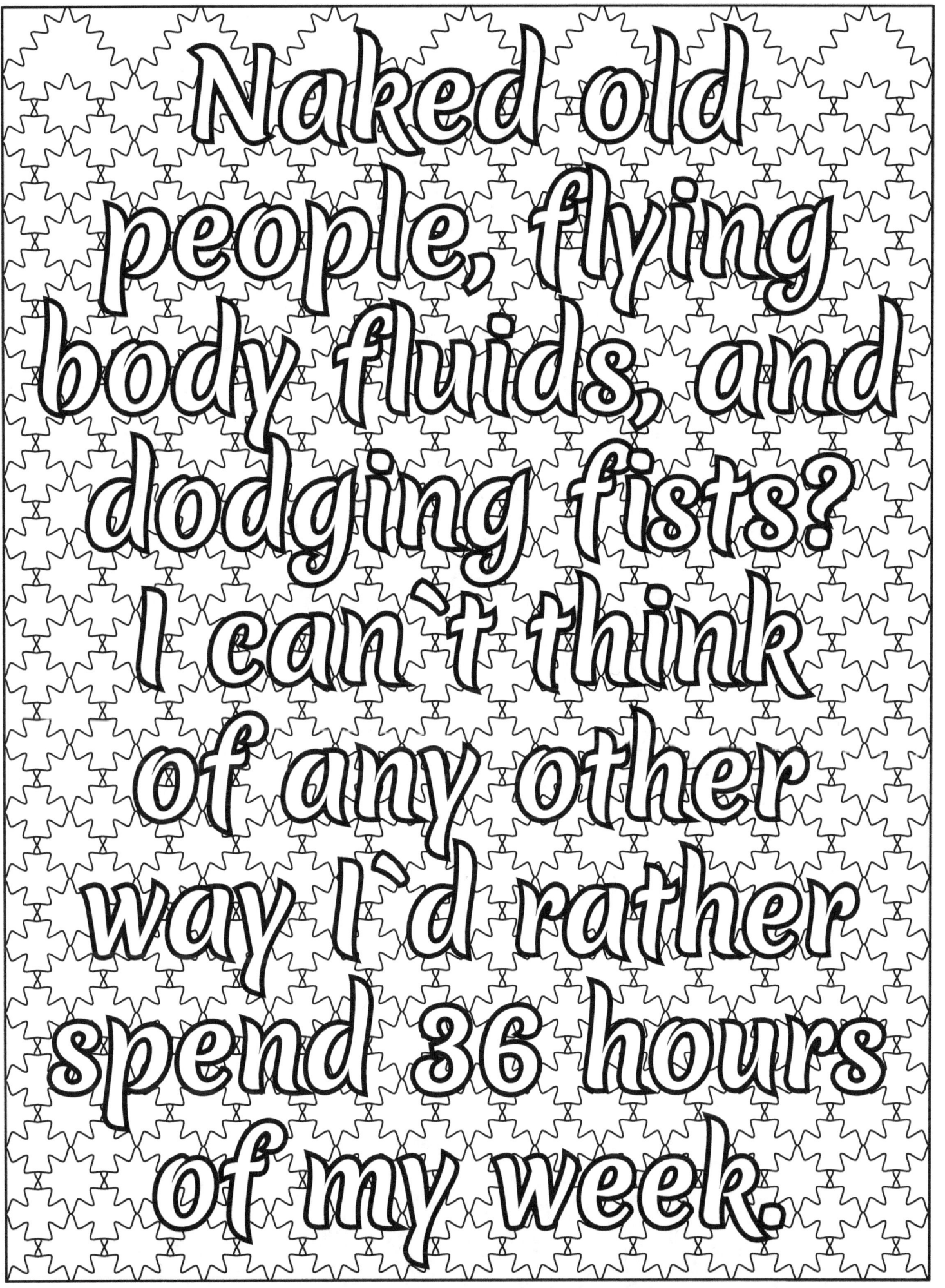

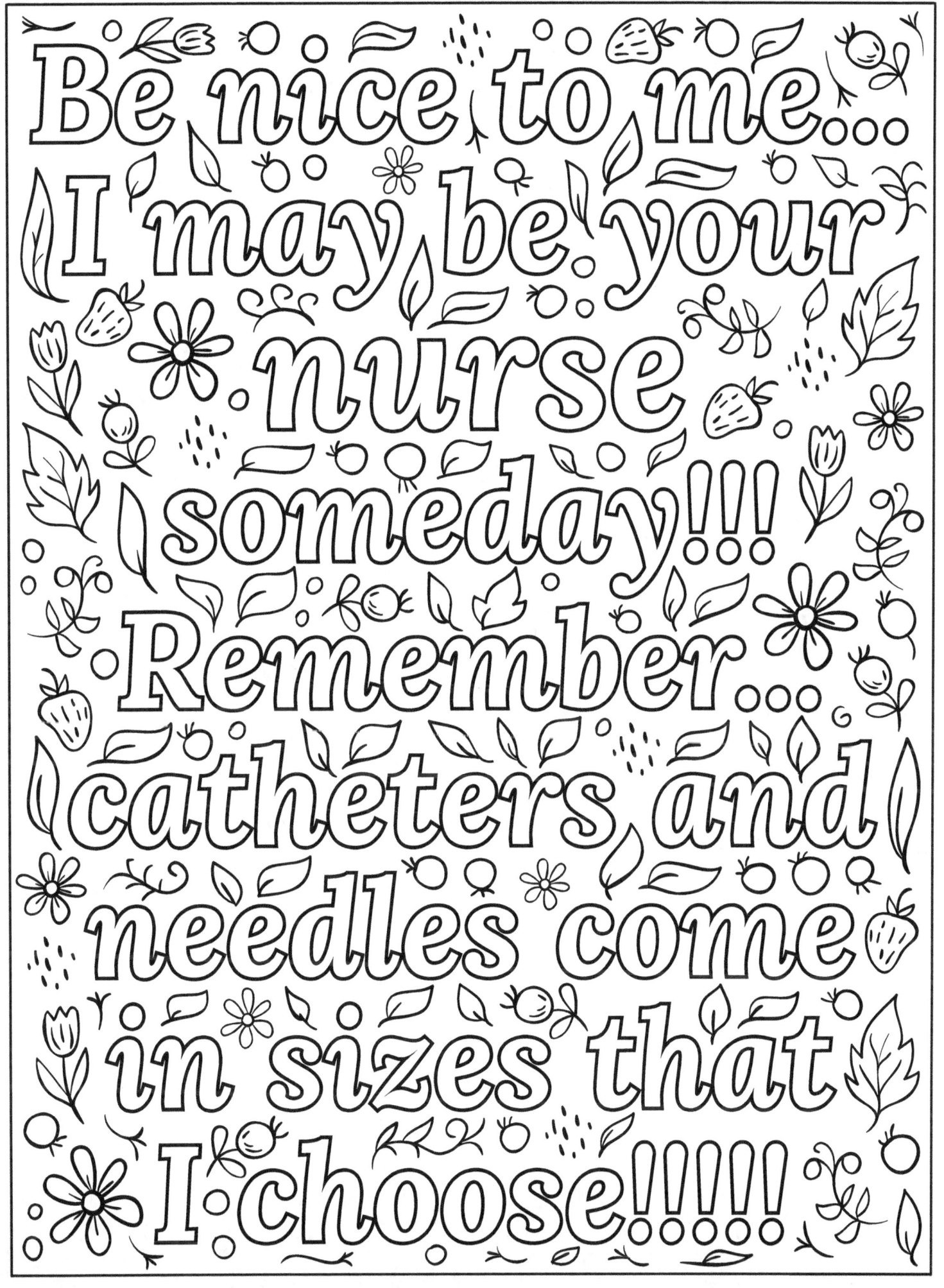

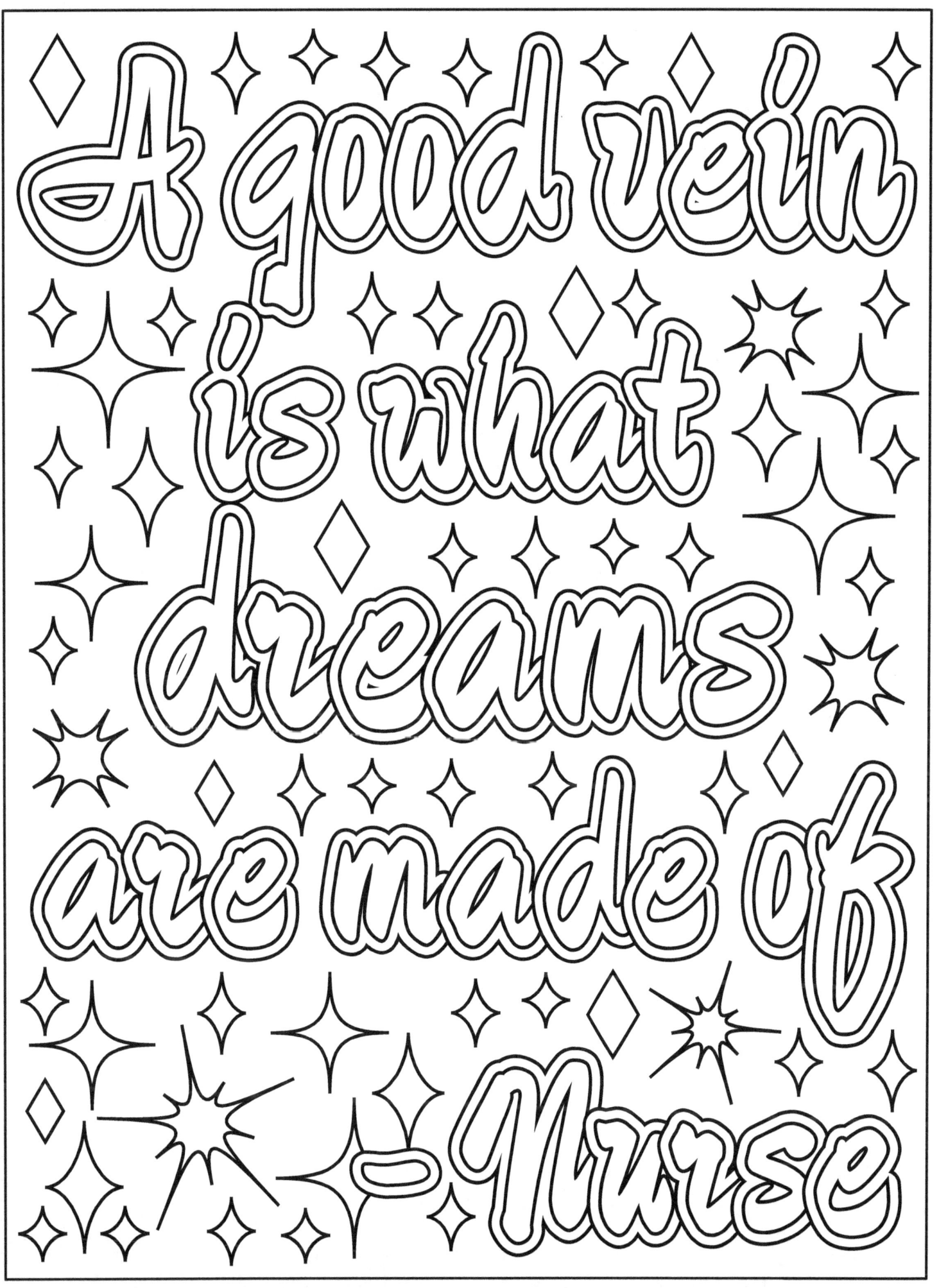

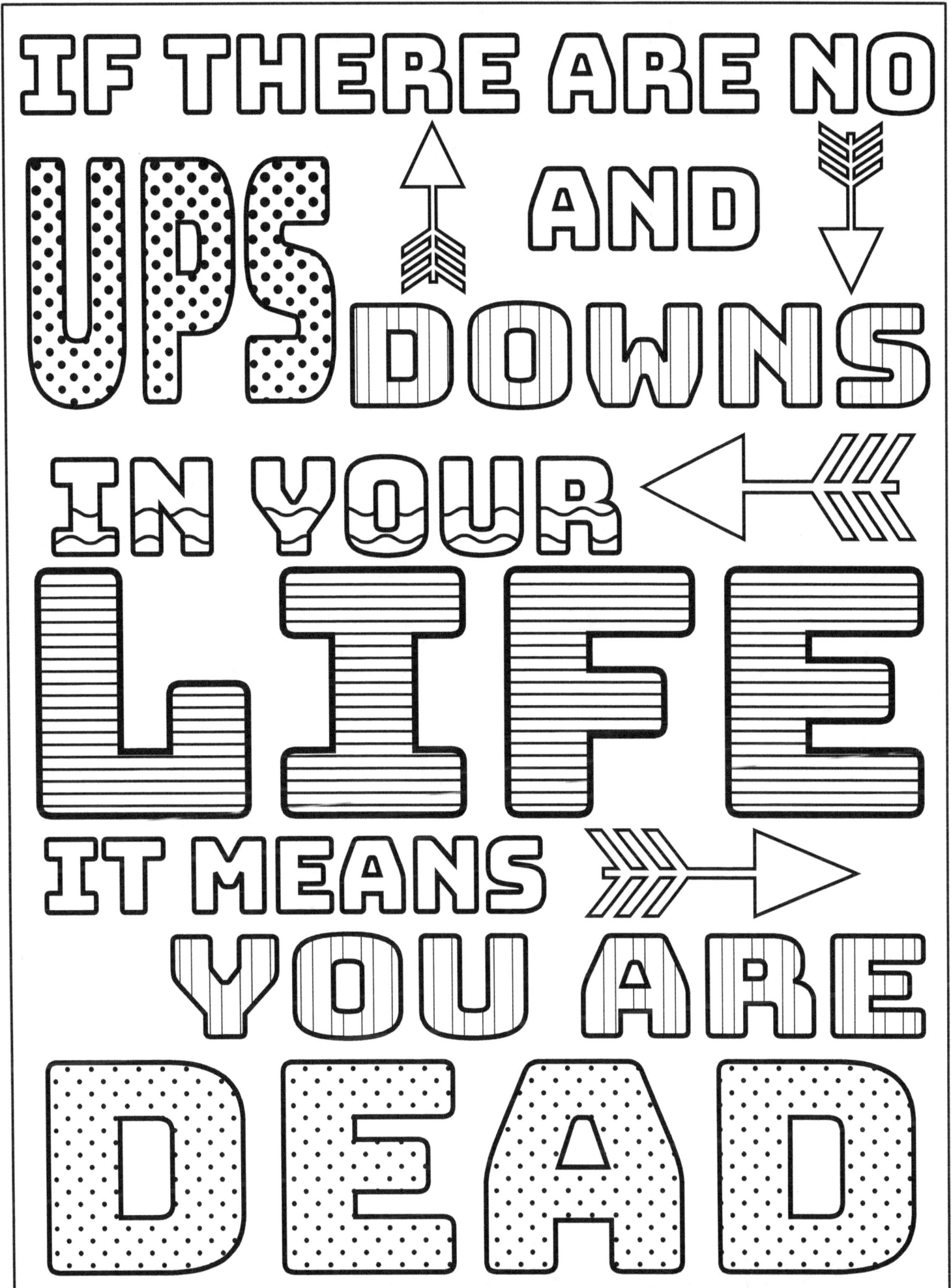

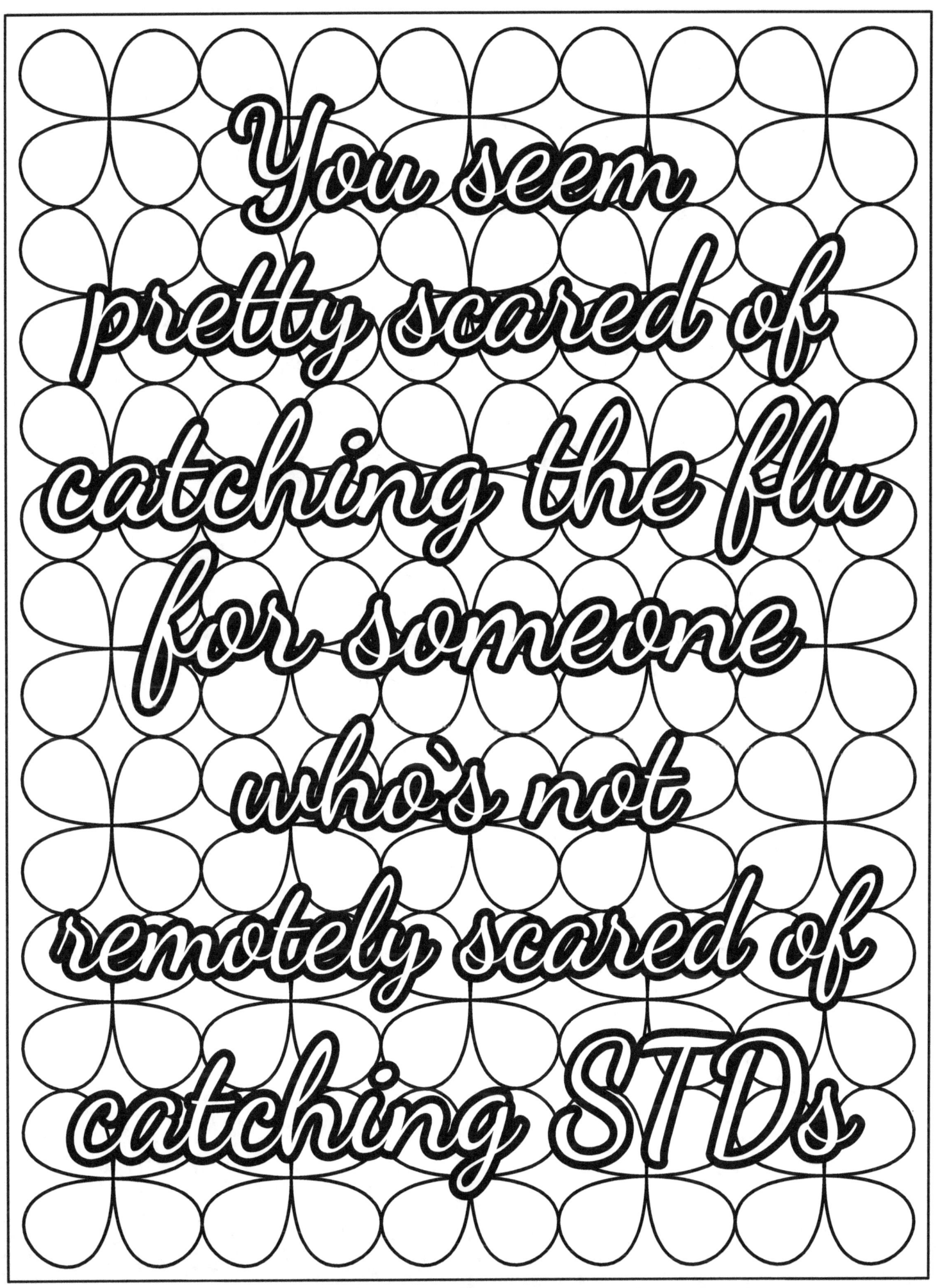

Most people dream of huge houses, nice cars and vacations. Not us.

We dream of normal work hours and a regular sleep schedule.

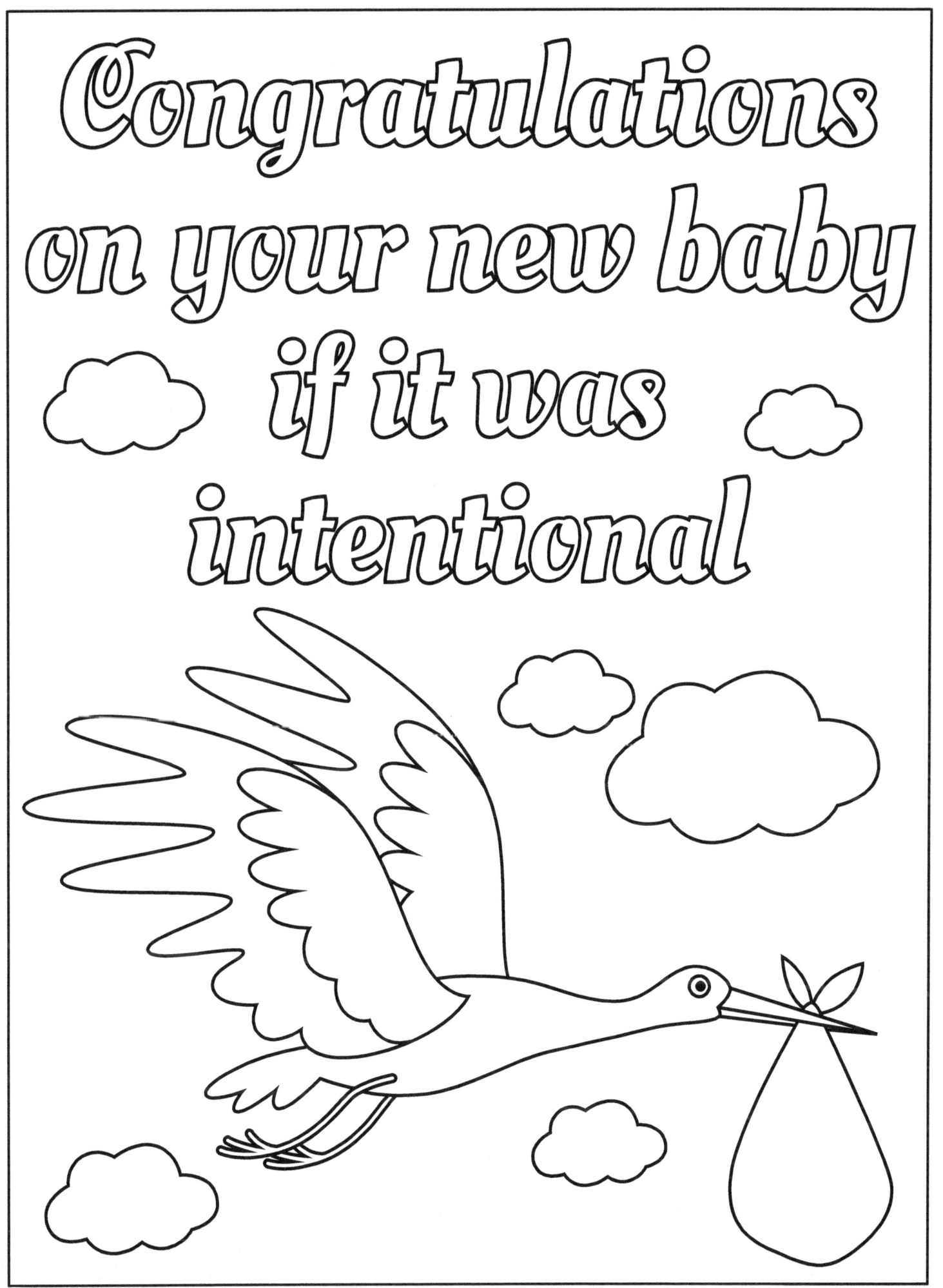

OMG!

A patient almost died in front of me today!! But then I counted to 10 and put my **scissors** back in my pocket. She never even knew.

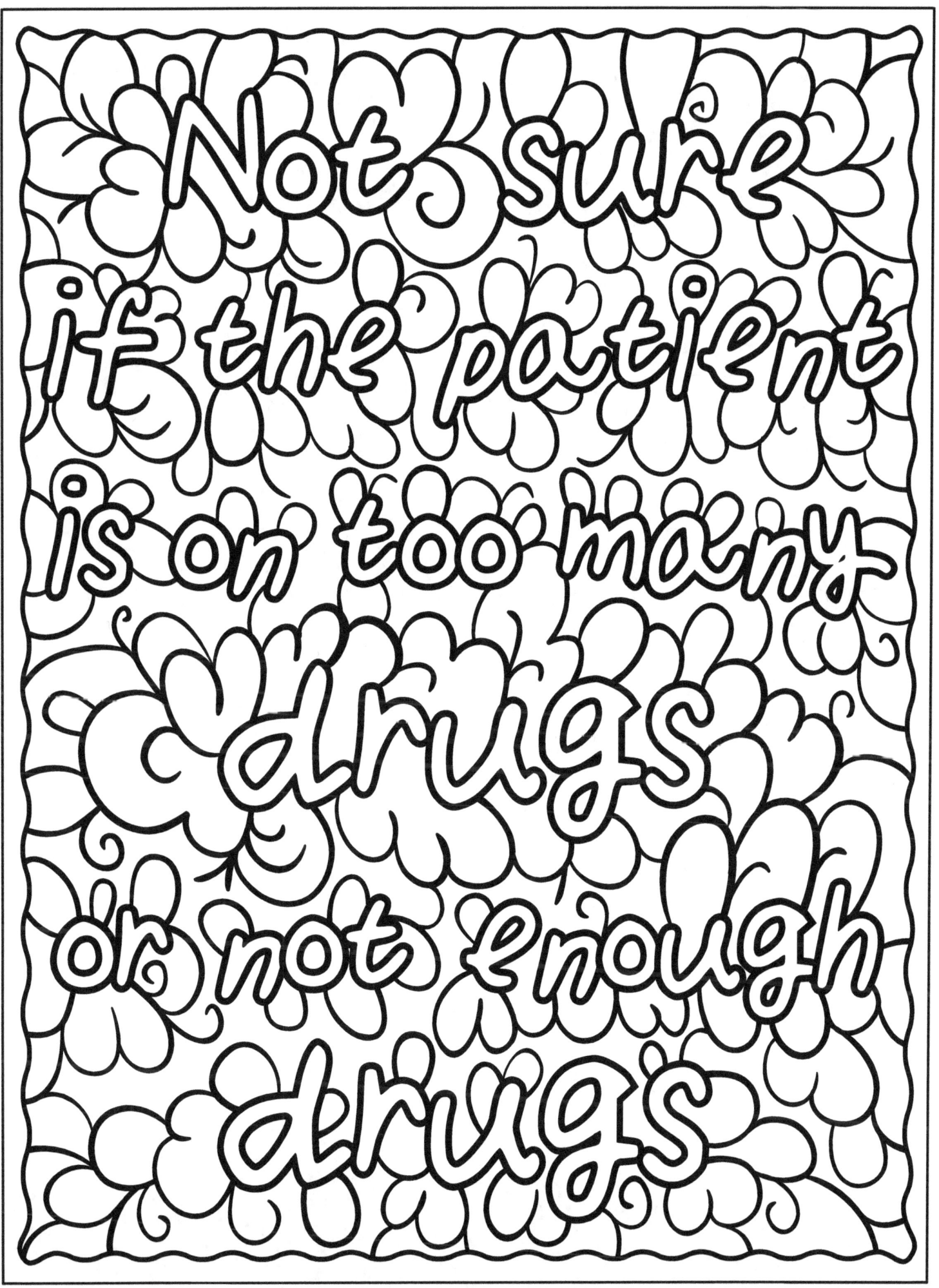

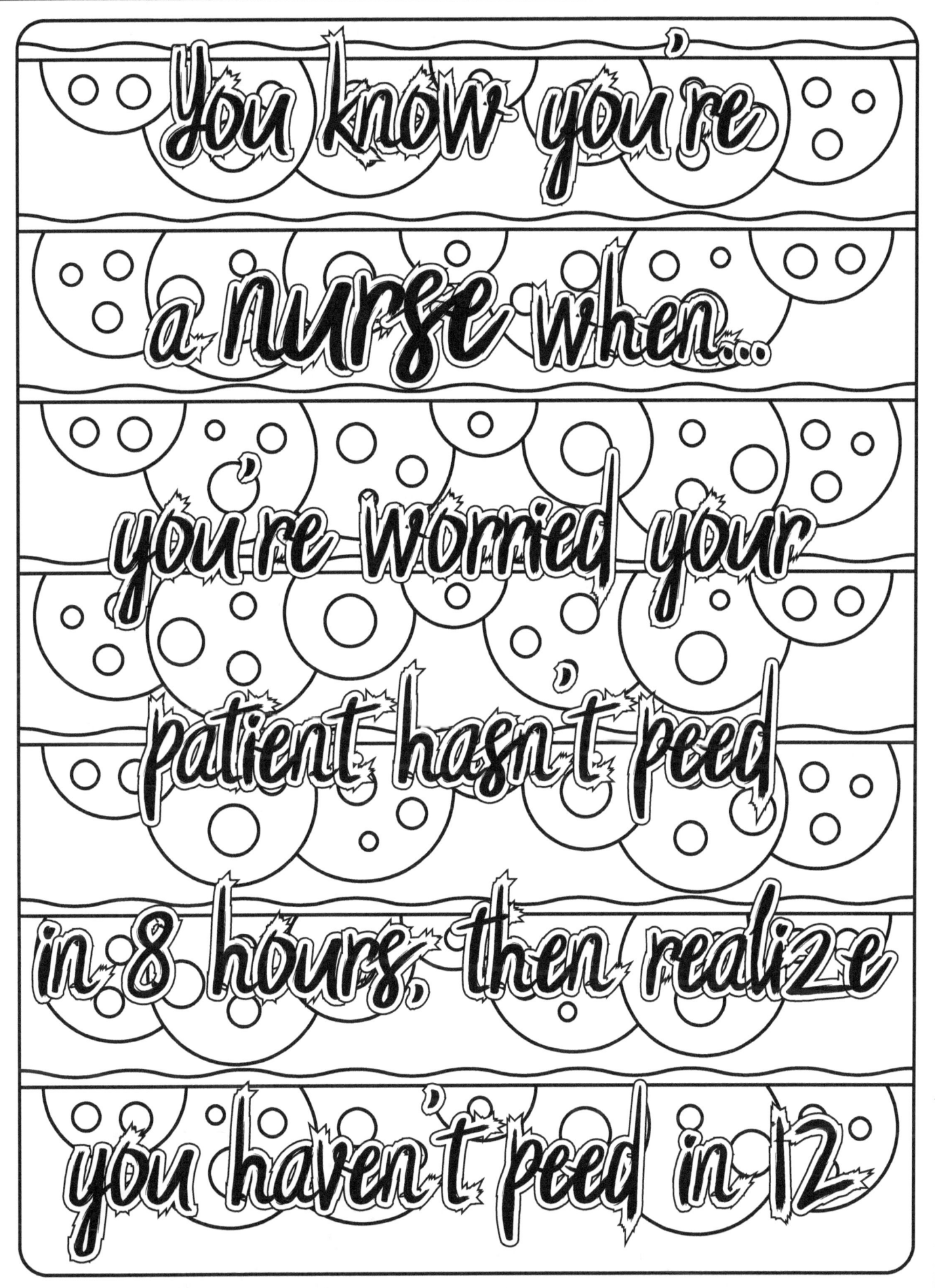

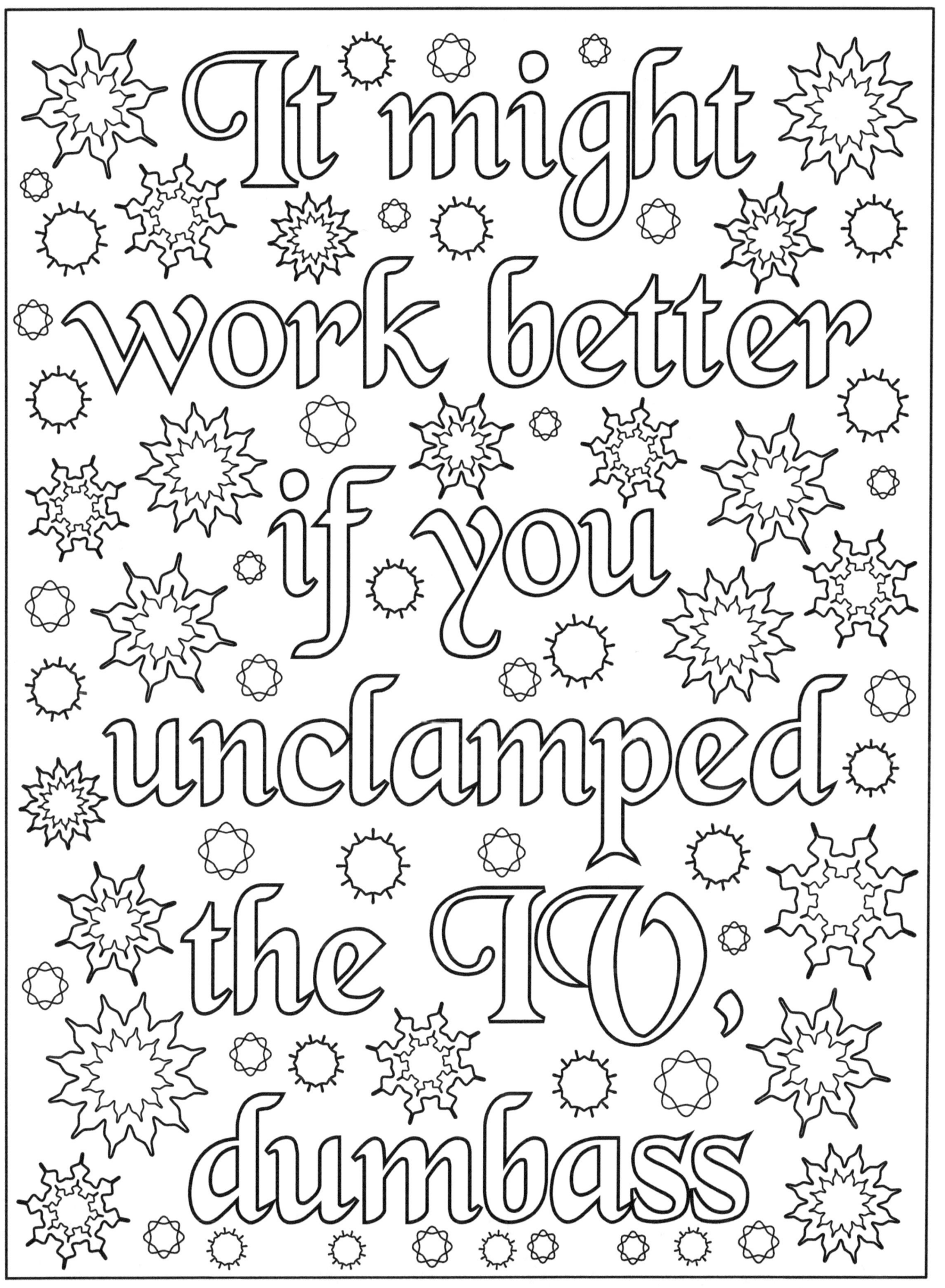

Quickest way to a man's heart? A bilateral incision on the upper left region of the sternum

IF EVERYONE'S MONITOR COULD STOP FUCKING BEEPING THAT'D BE GREAT

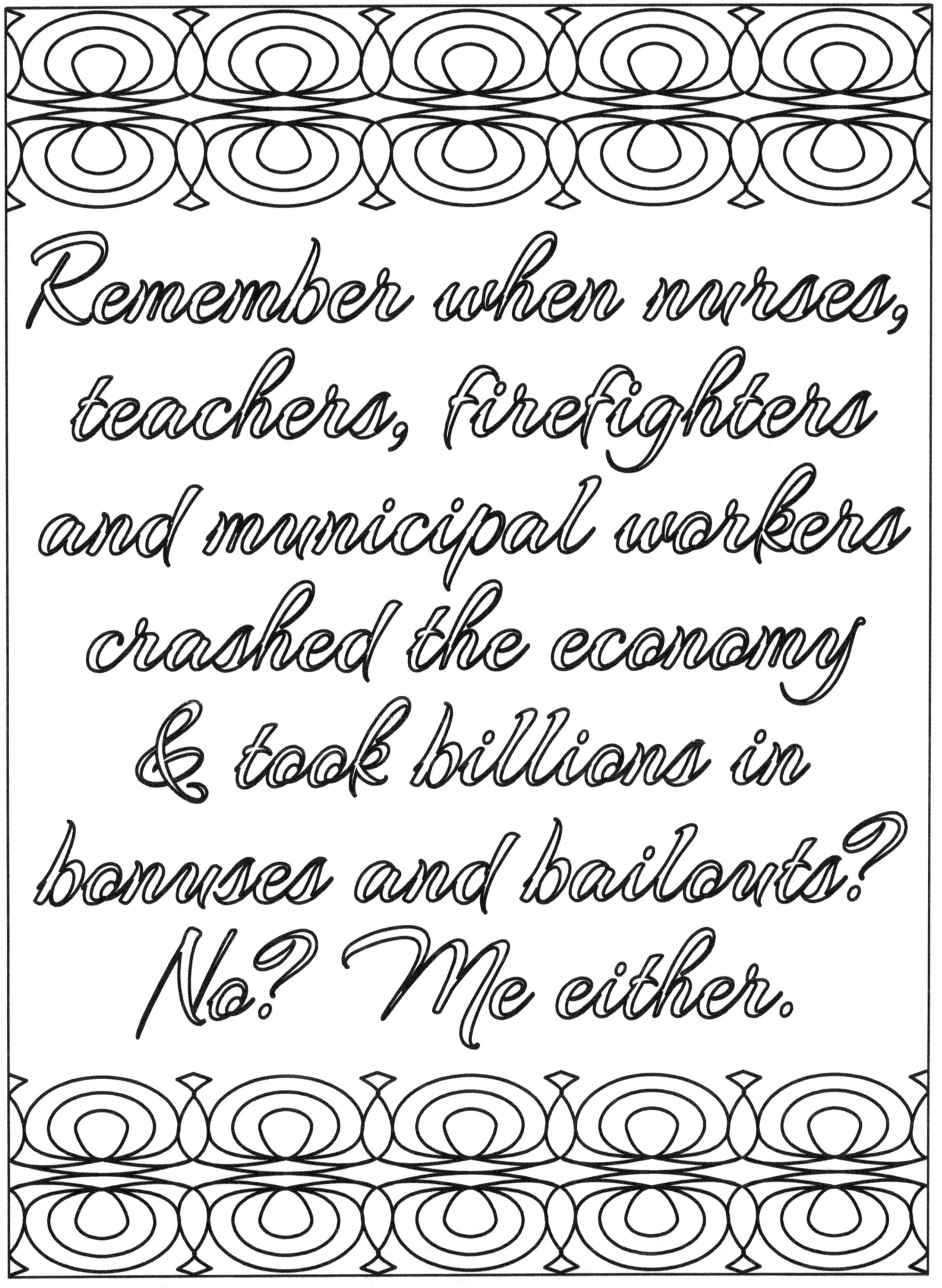

You know that feeling when you meet someone and your heart skips a beat?

Yeah, that's arrhythmia. You can die from that.

YES, I CHARTED THAT I CHARTED WHAT I PREVIOUSLY CHARTED. WAIT, HOLD ON. I HAVE TO CHART THAT I TOLD YOU ABOUT MY CHARTING.

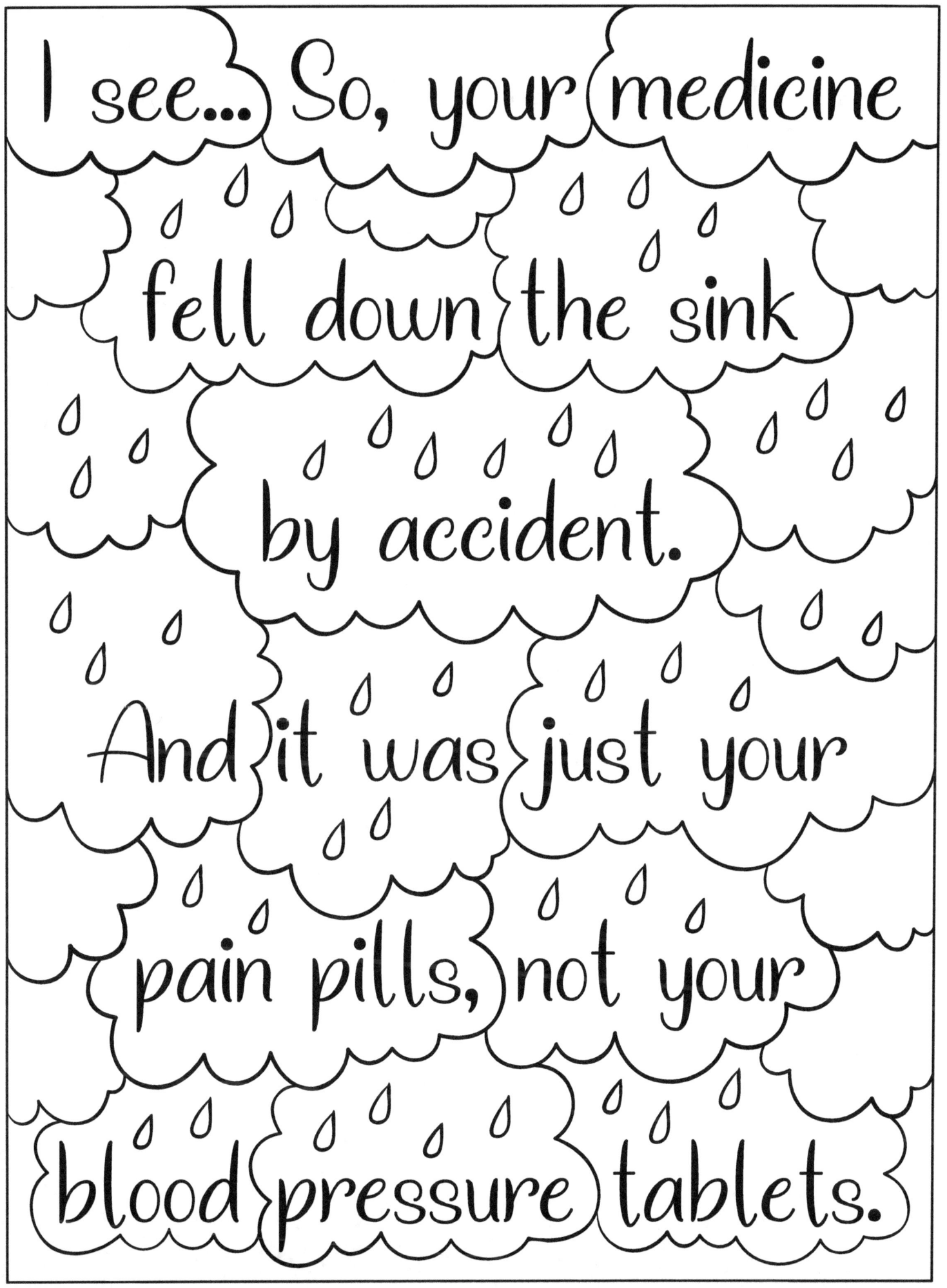

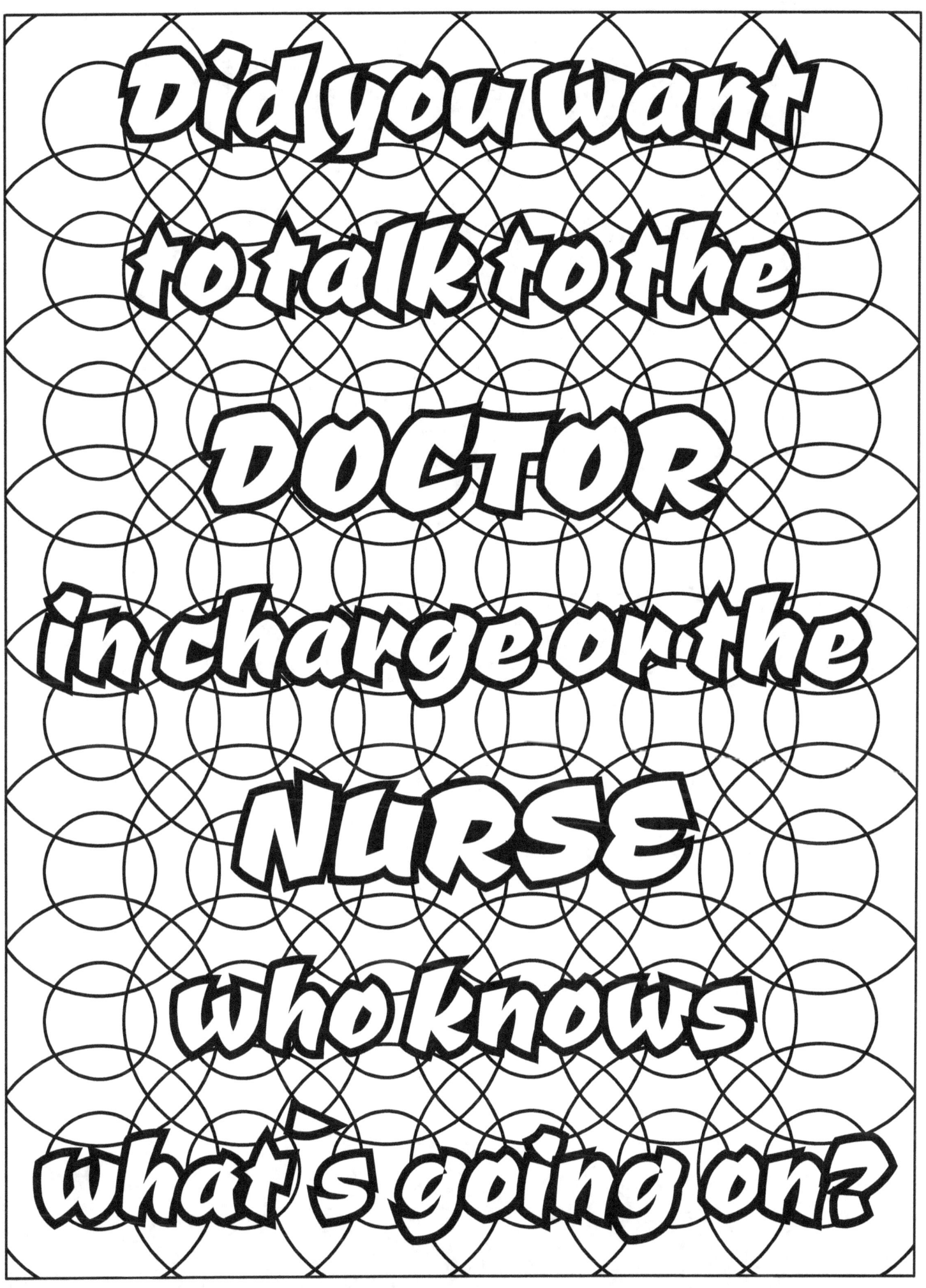

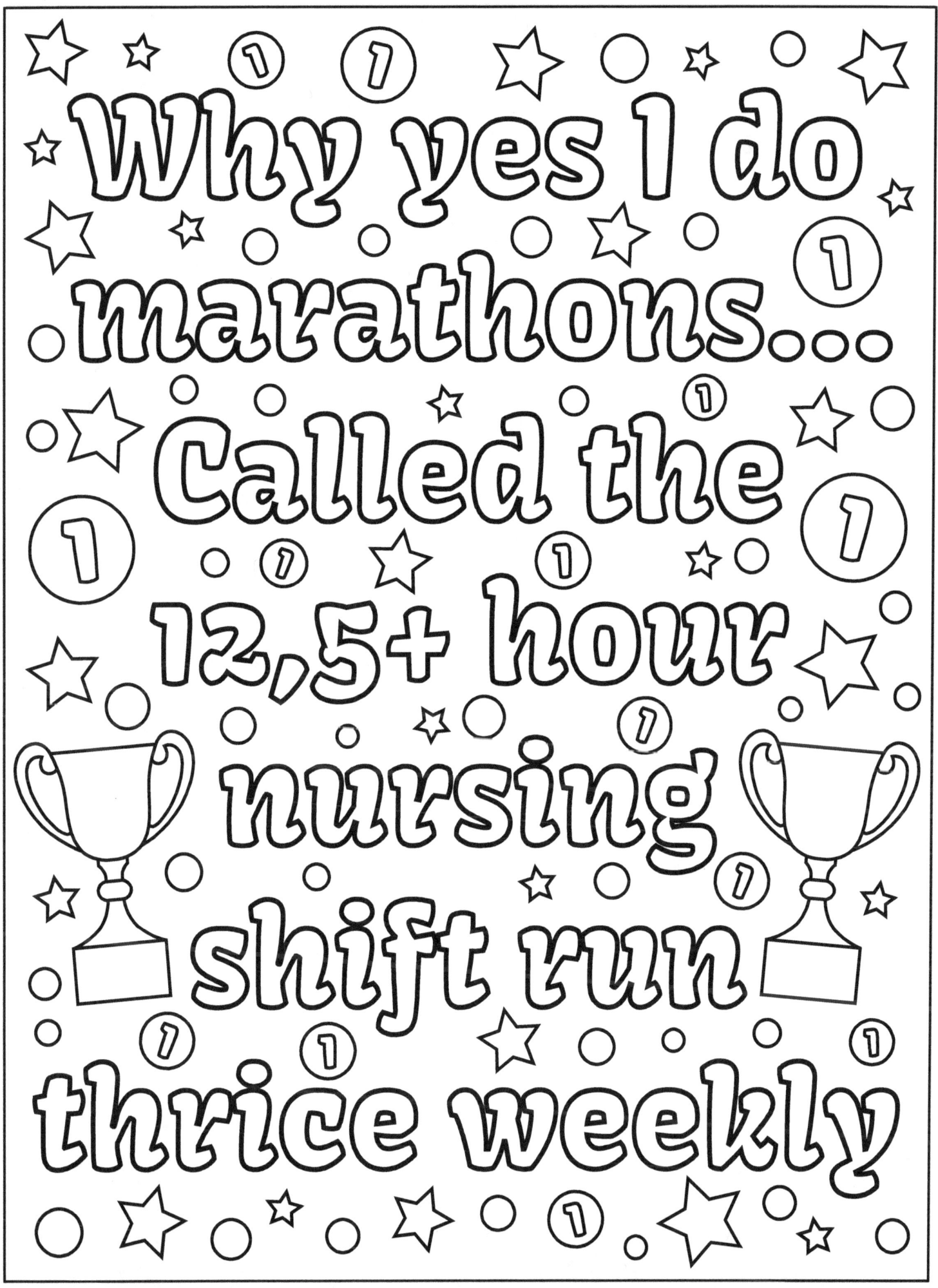

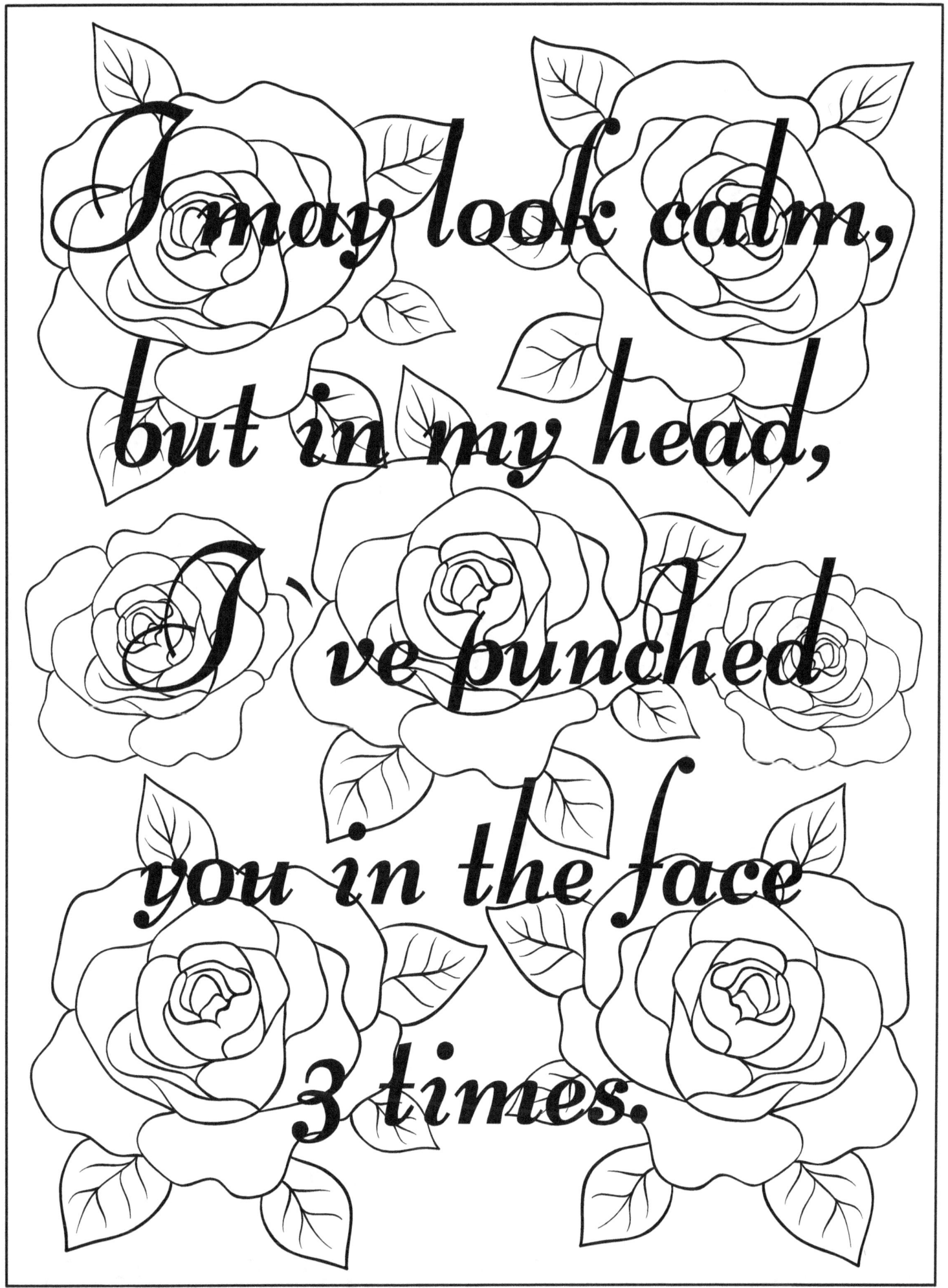

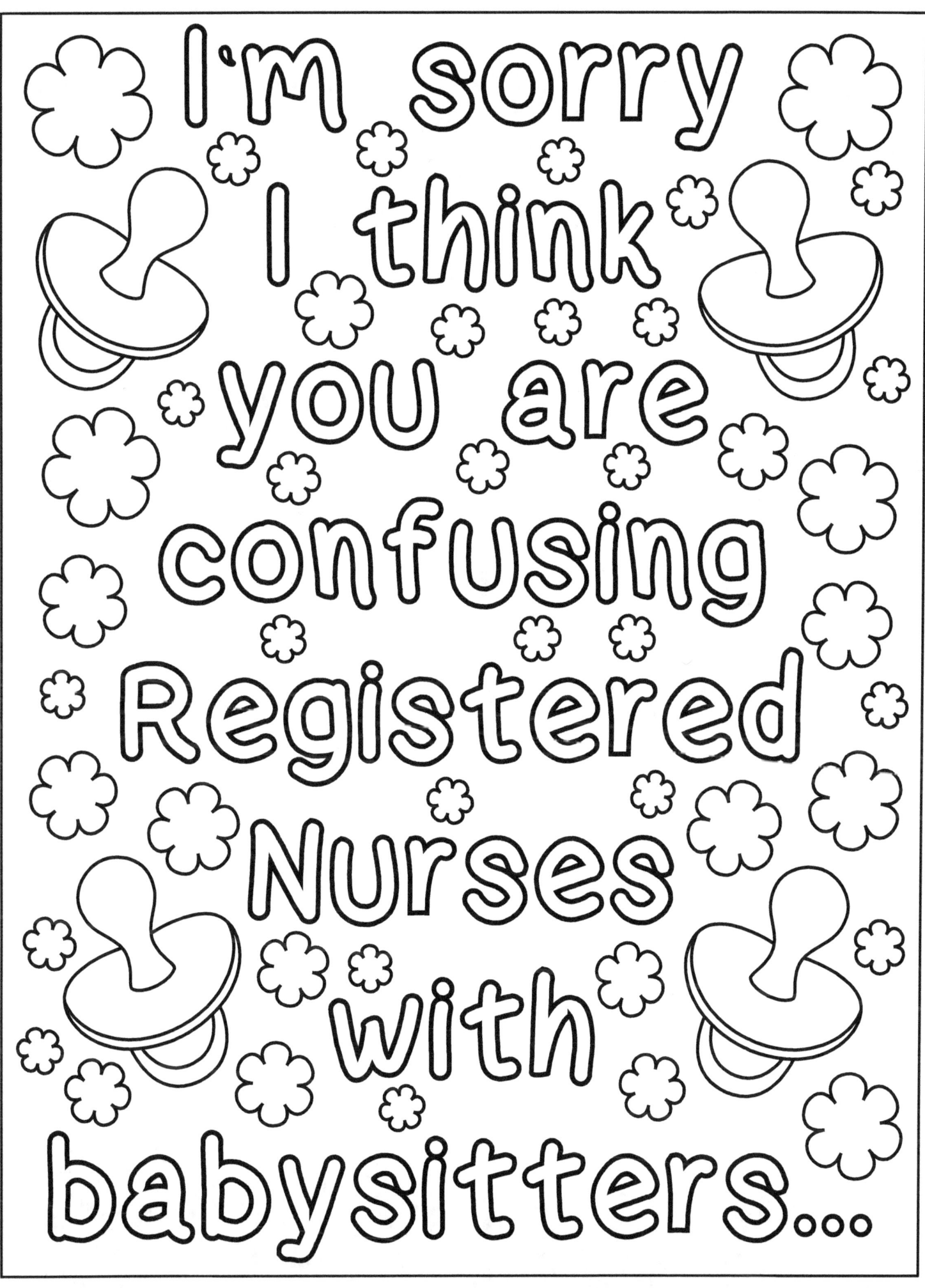

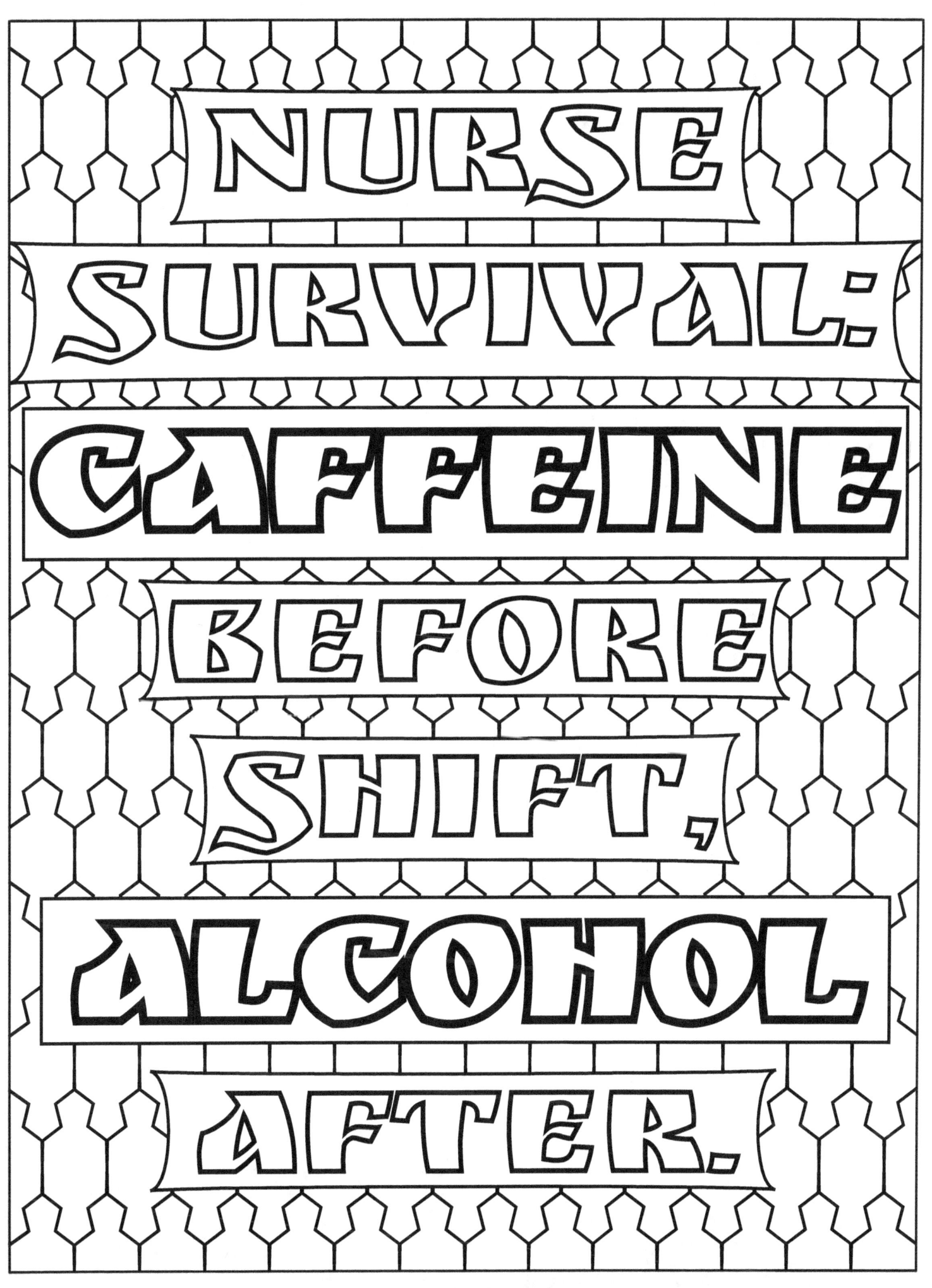

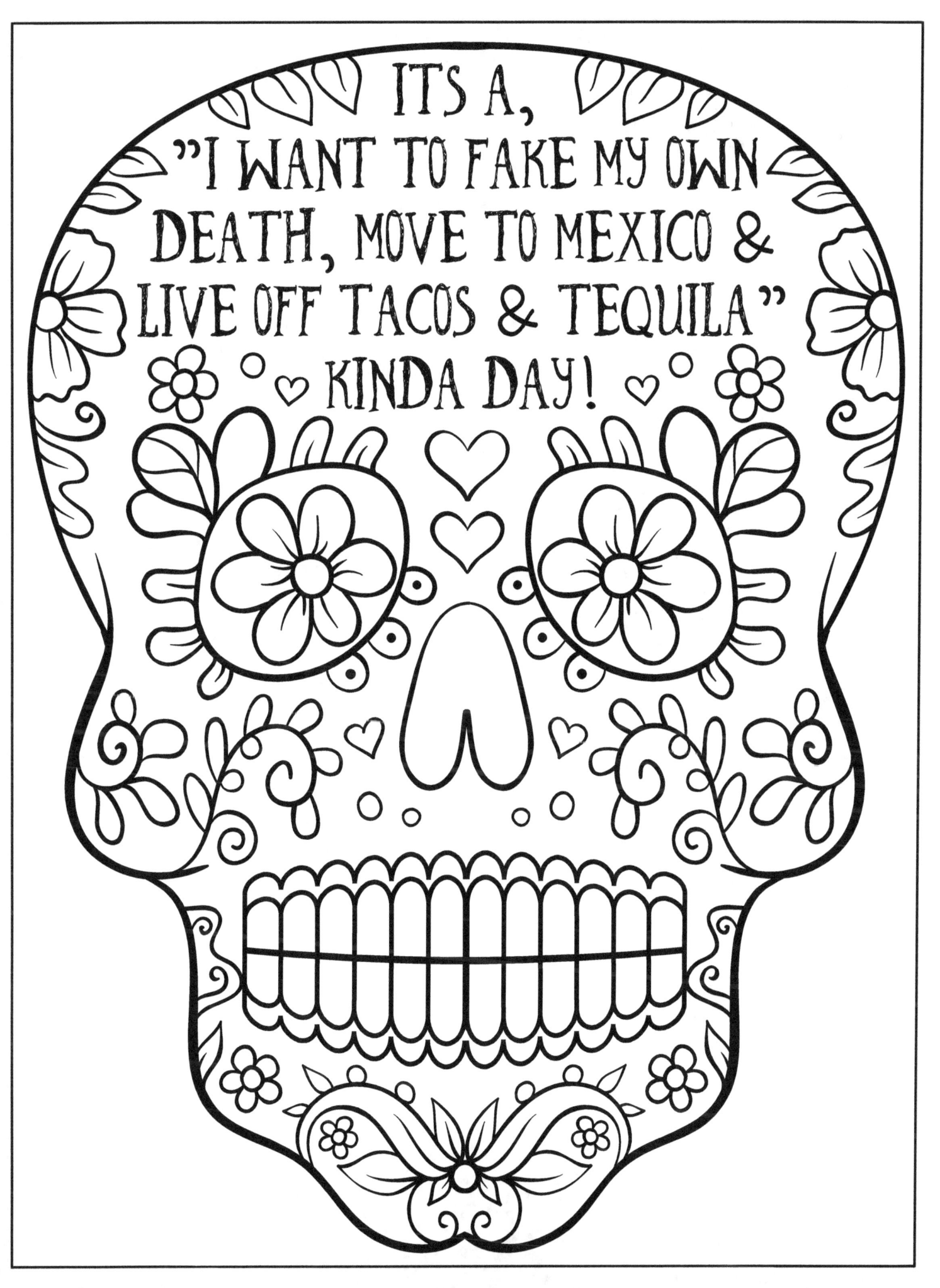

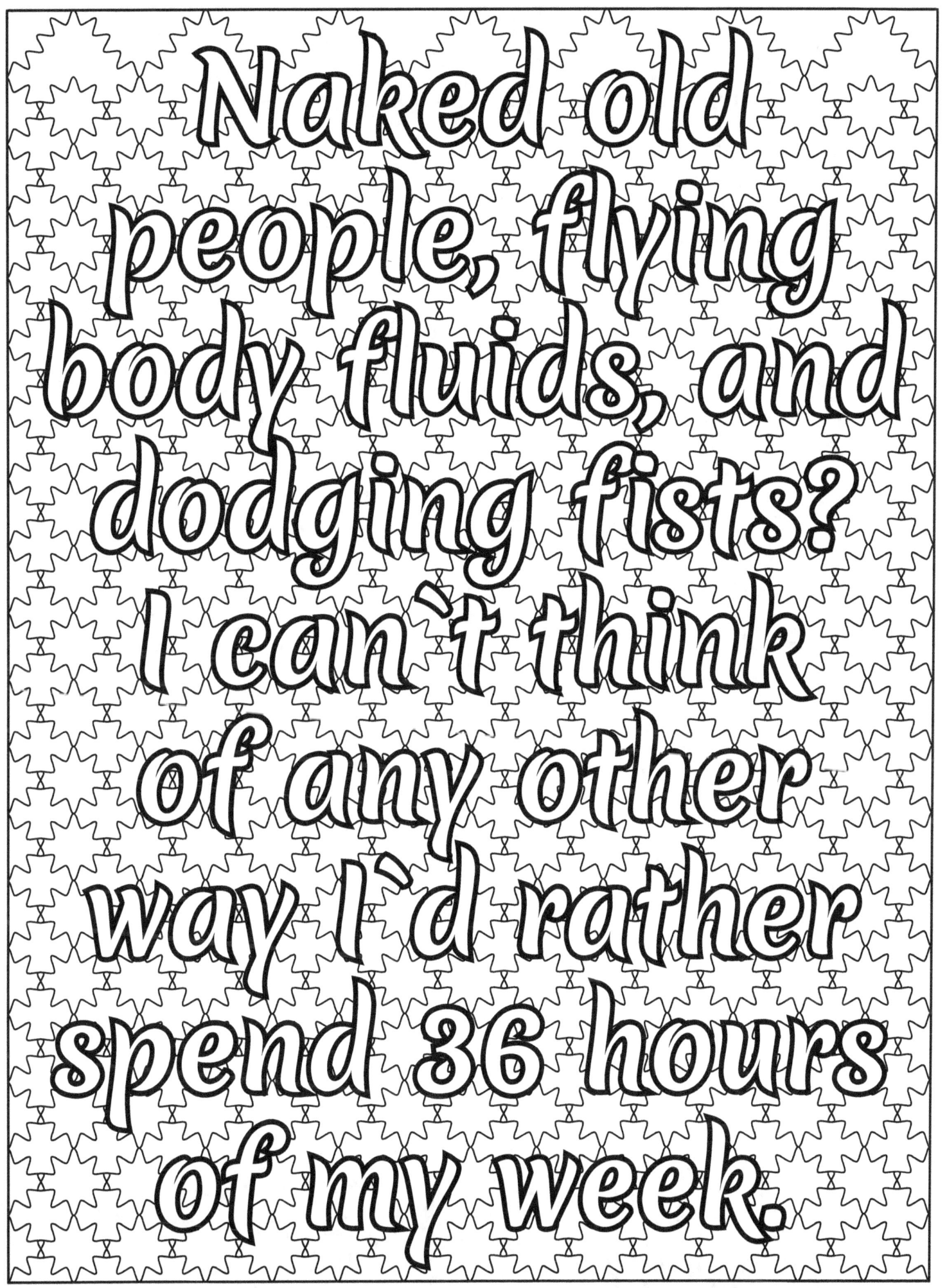

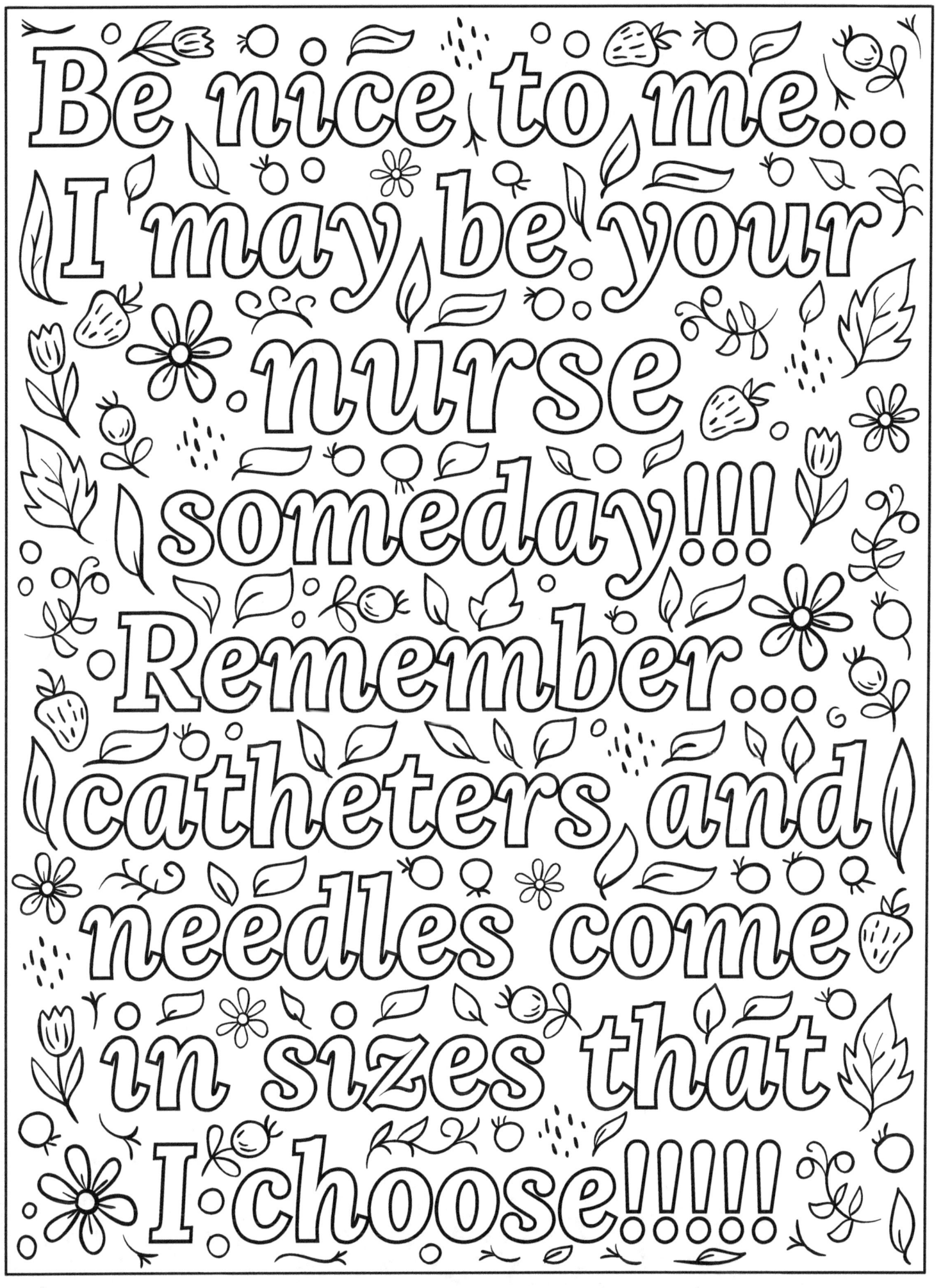

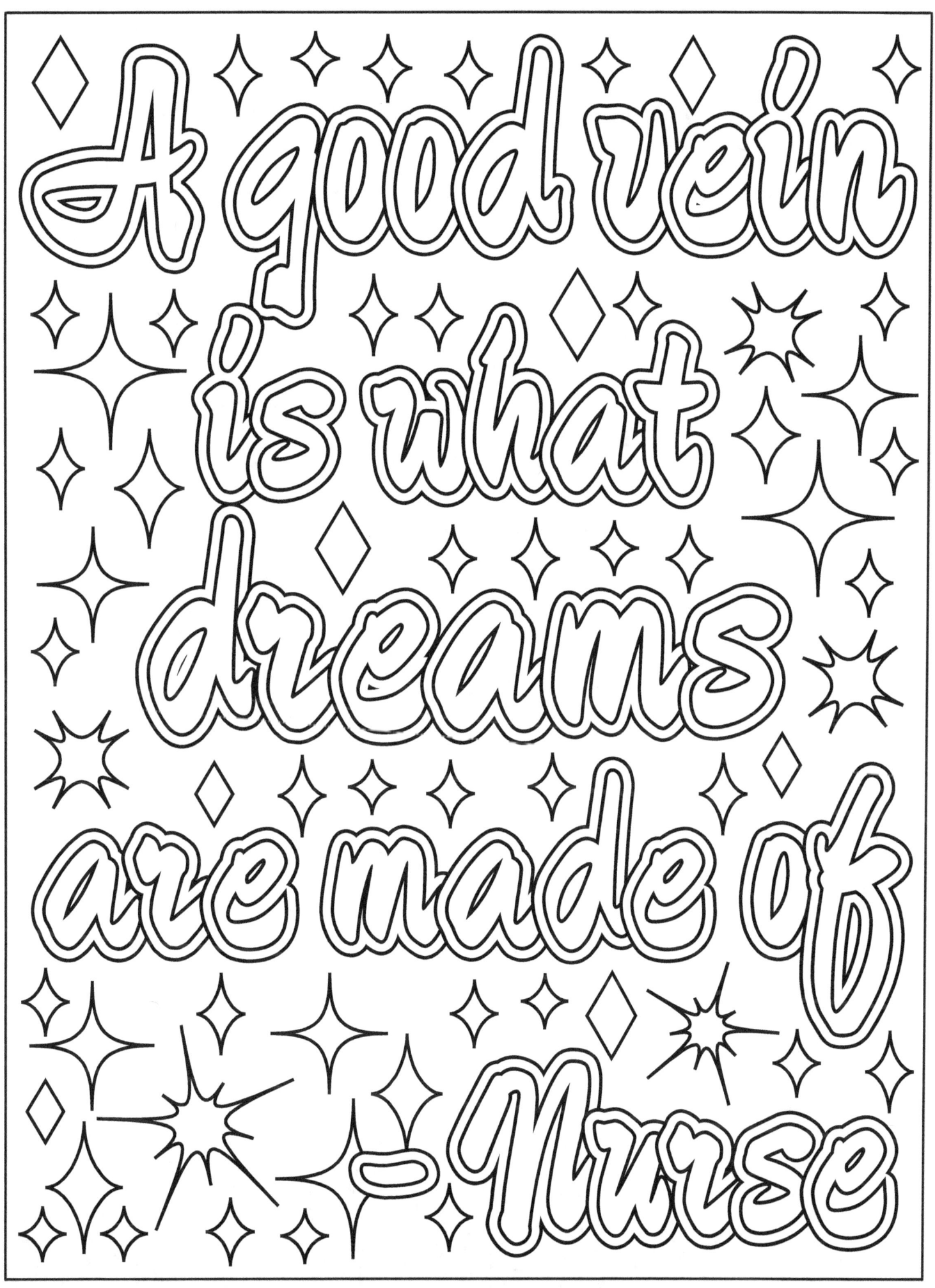

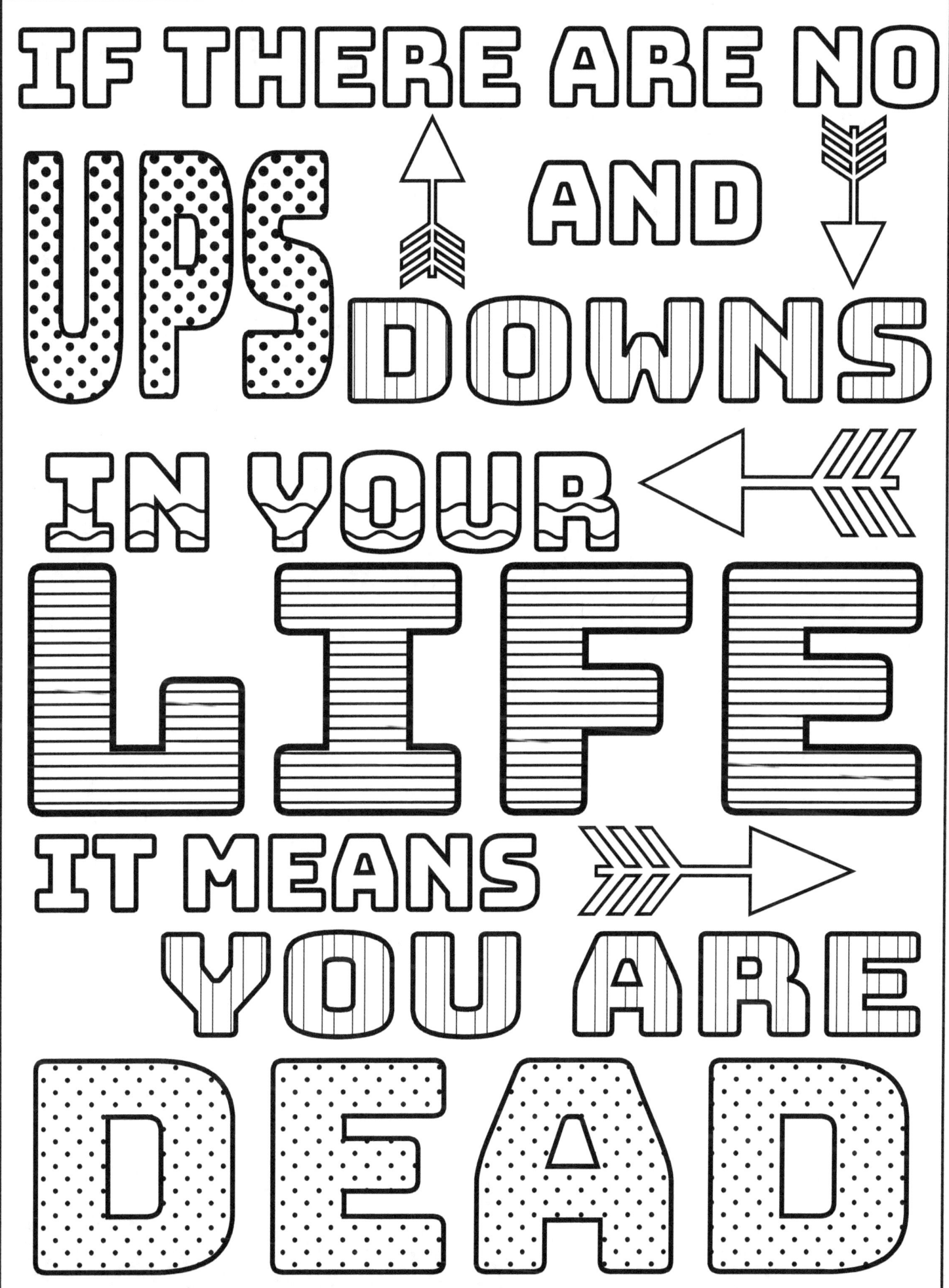

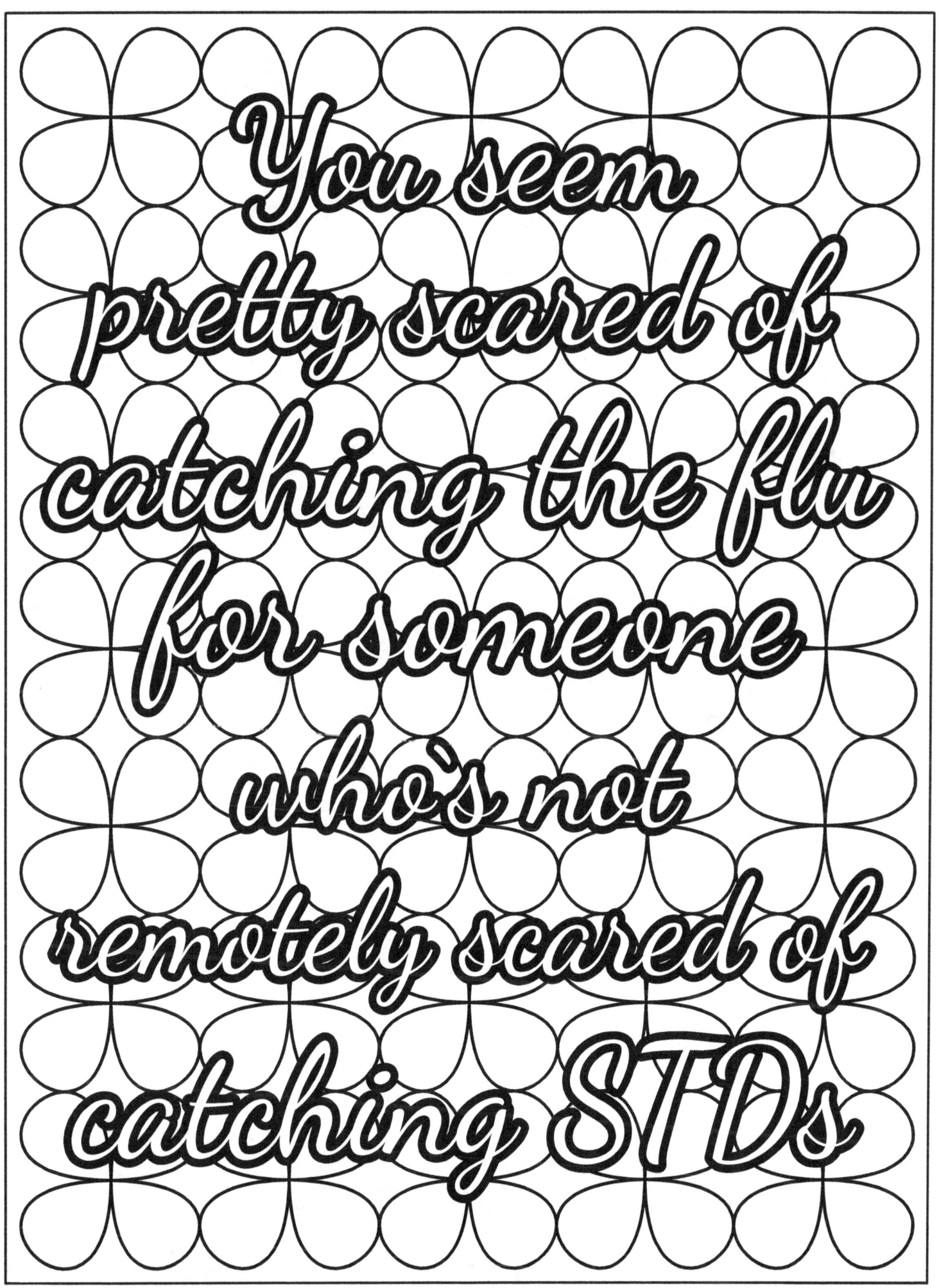

Most people dream of huge houses, nice cars and vacations. Not us.

We dream of normal work hours and a regular sleep schedule.

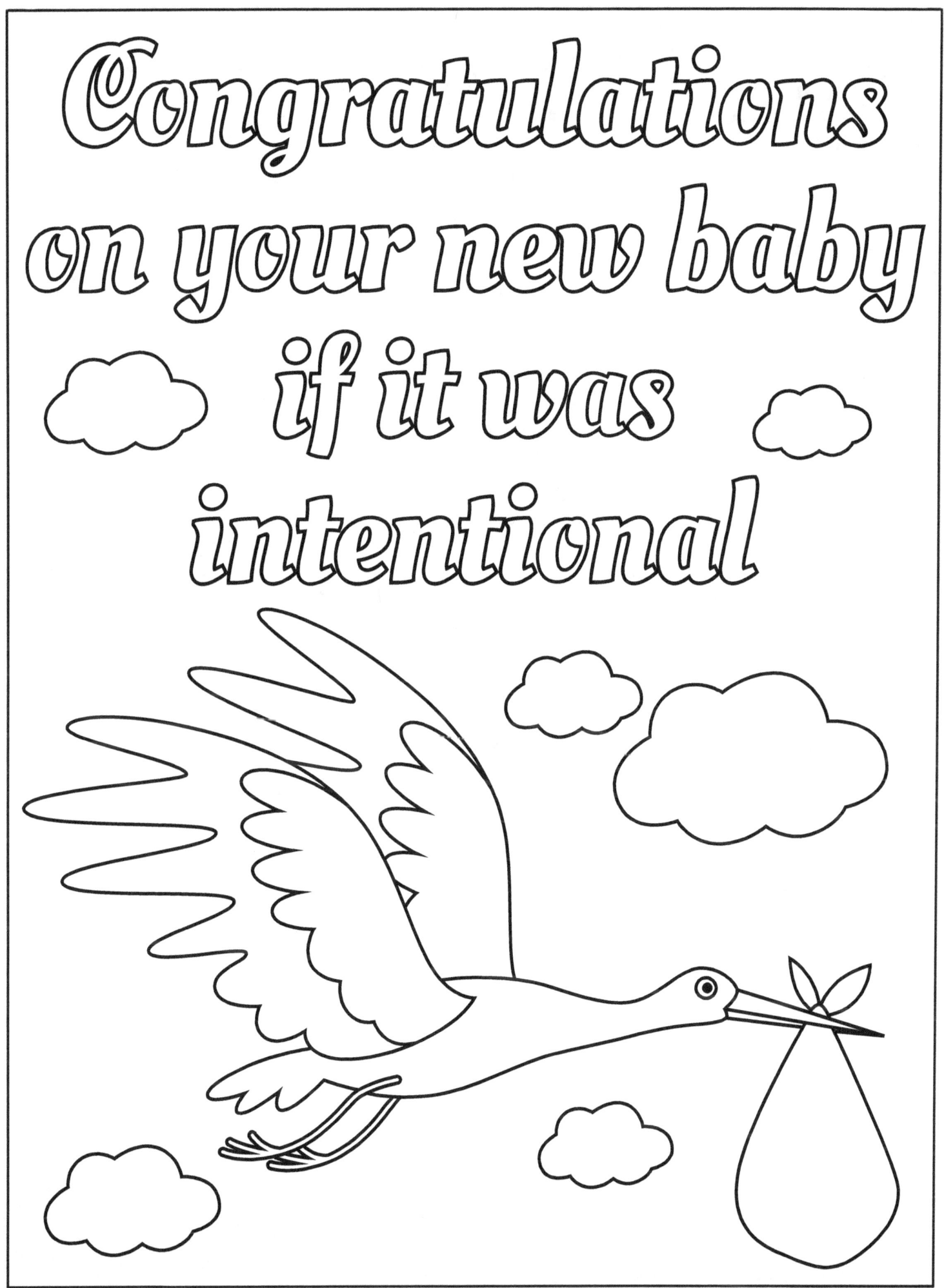

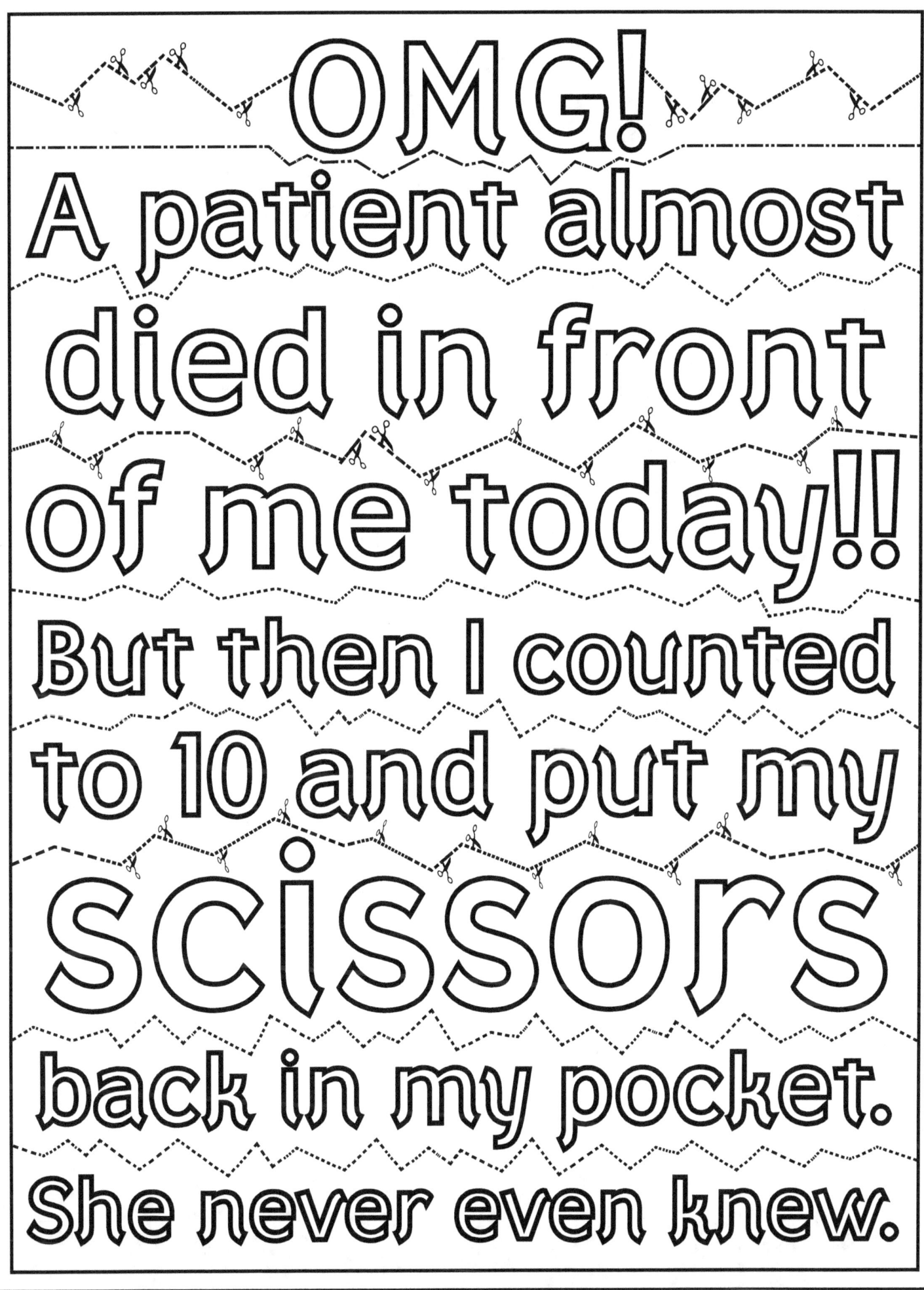

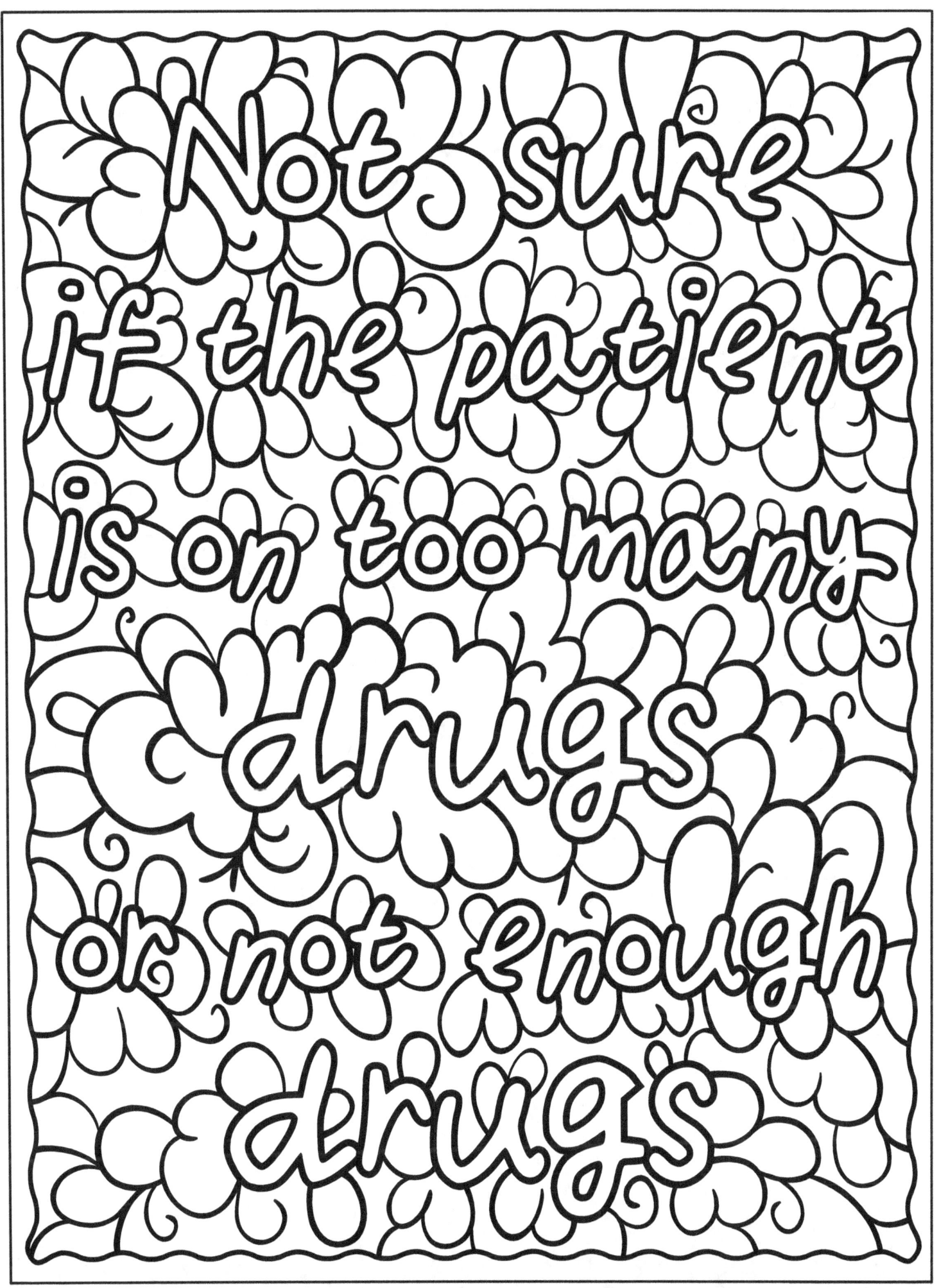

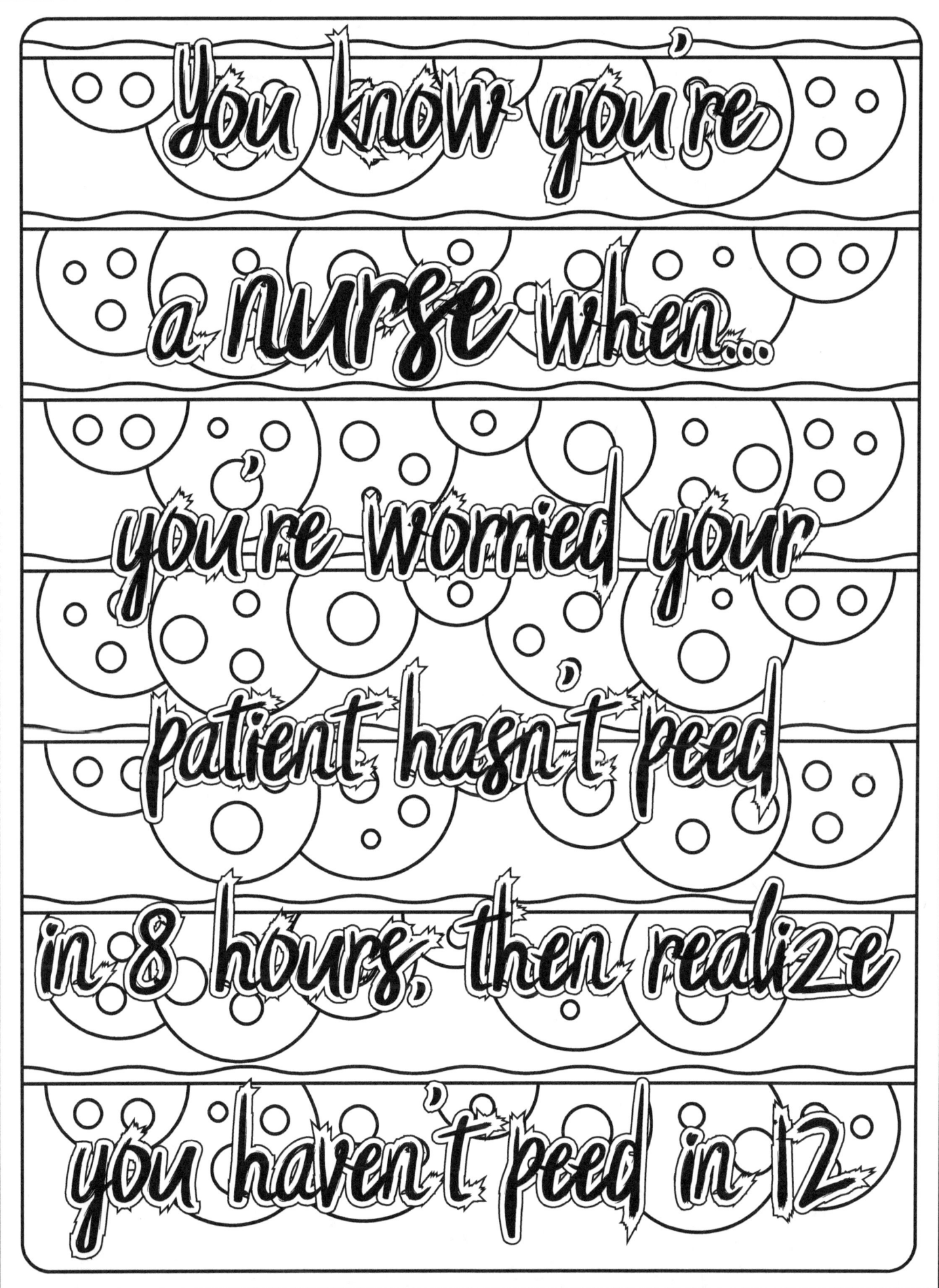

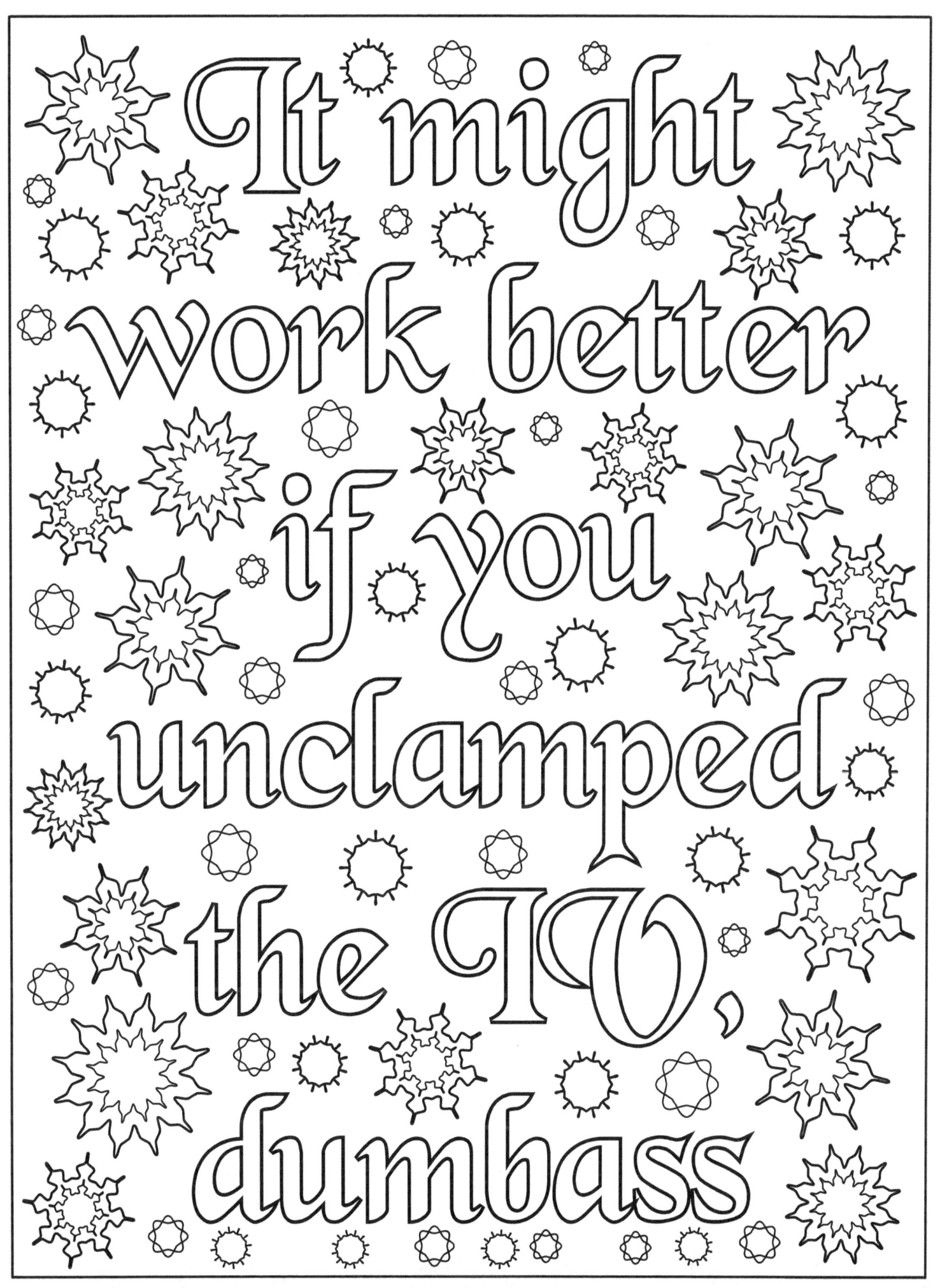

Quickest way to a man's heart? A bilateral incision on the upper left region of the sternum

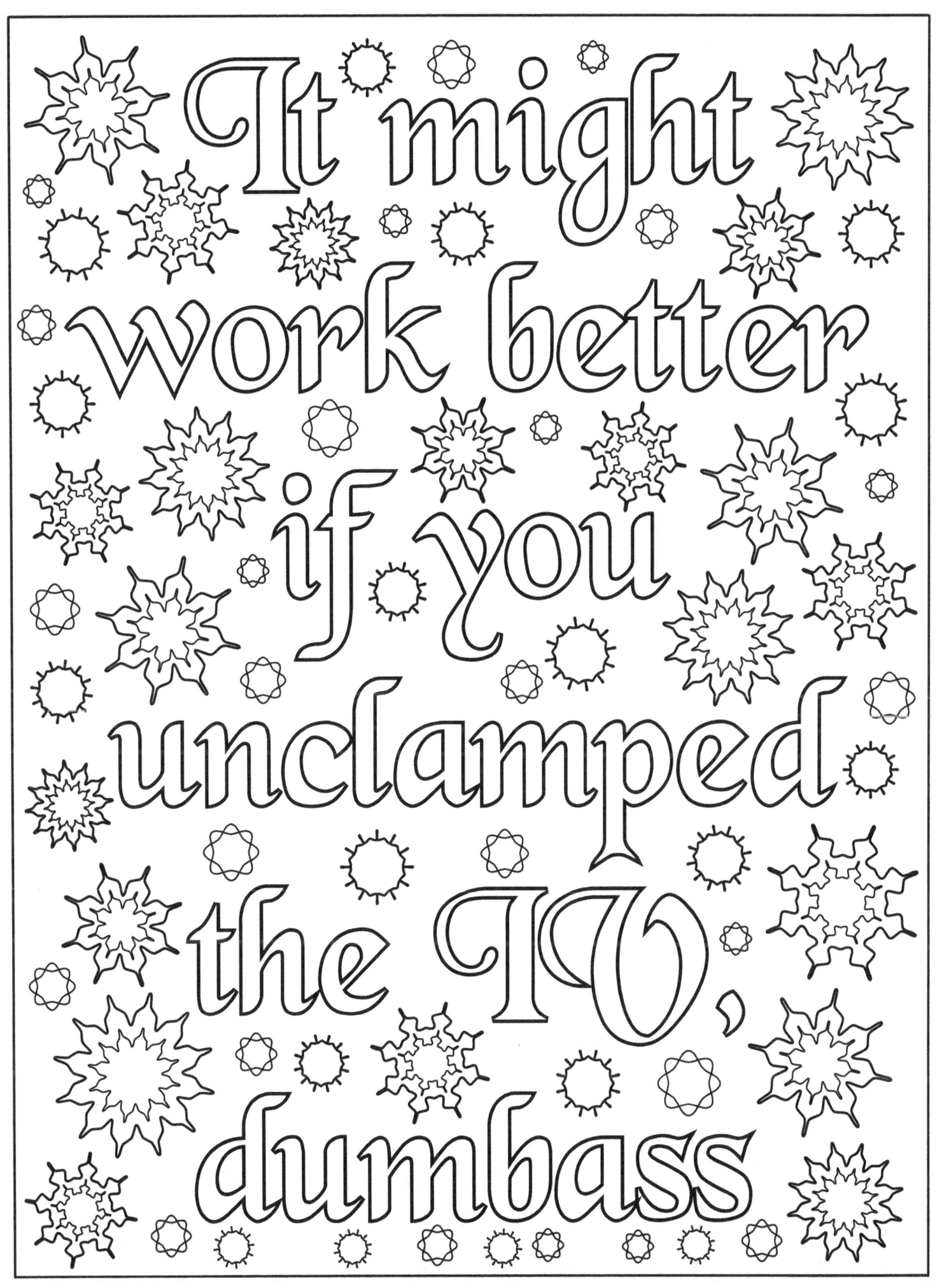

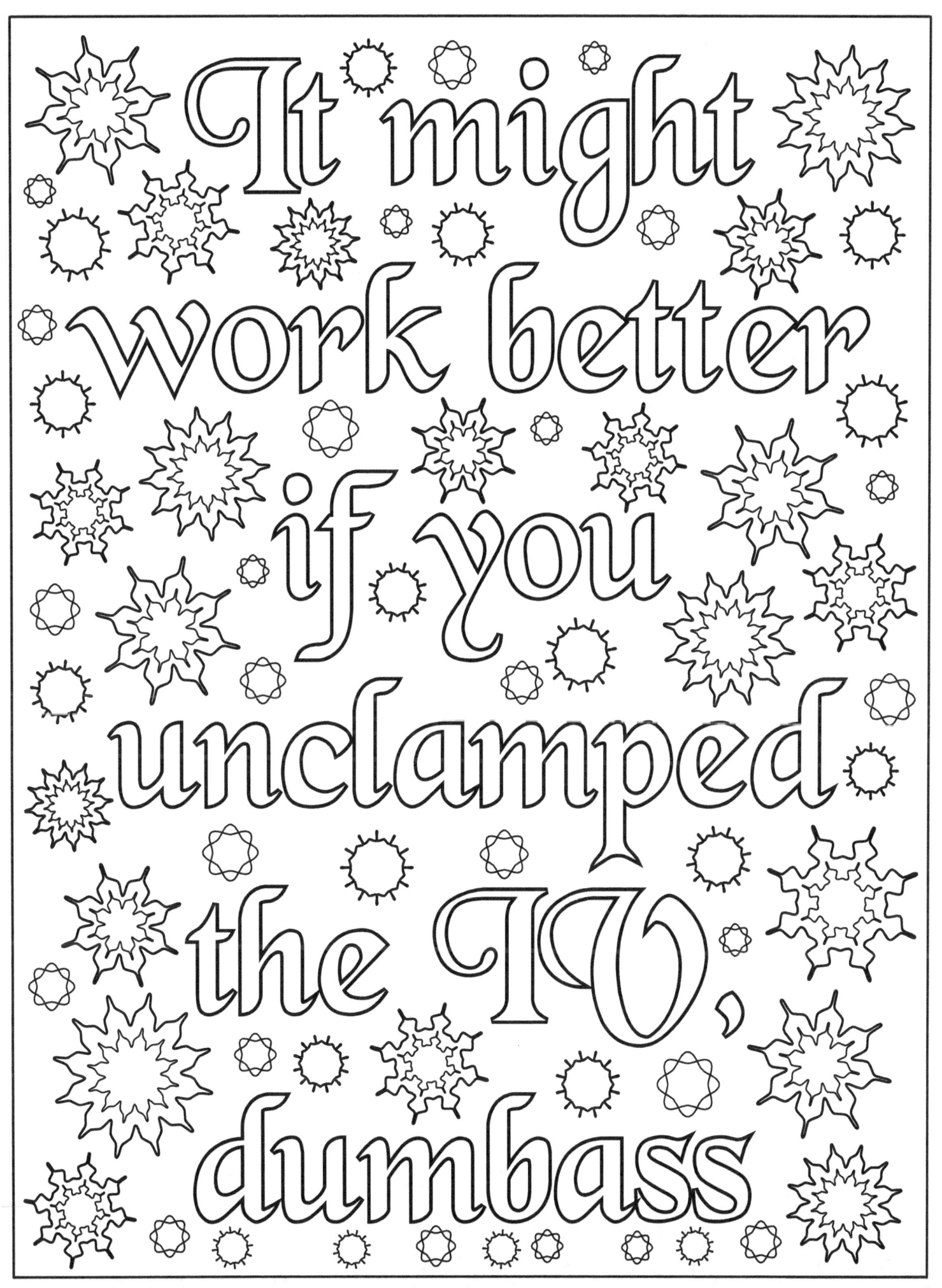

IF EVERYONE'S MONITOR COULD STOP FUCKING BEEPING THAT'D BE GREAT

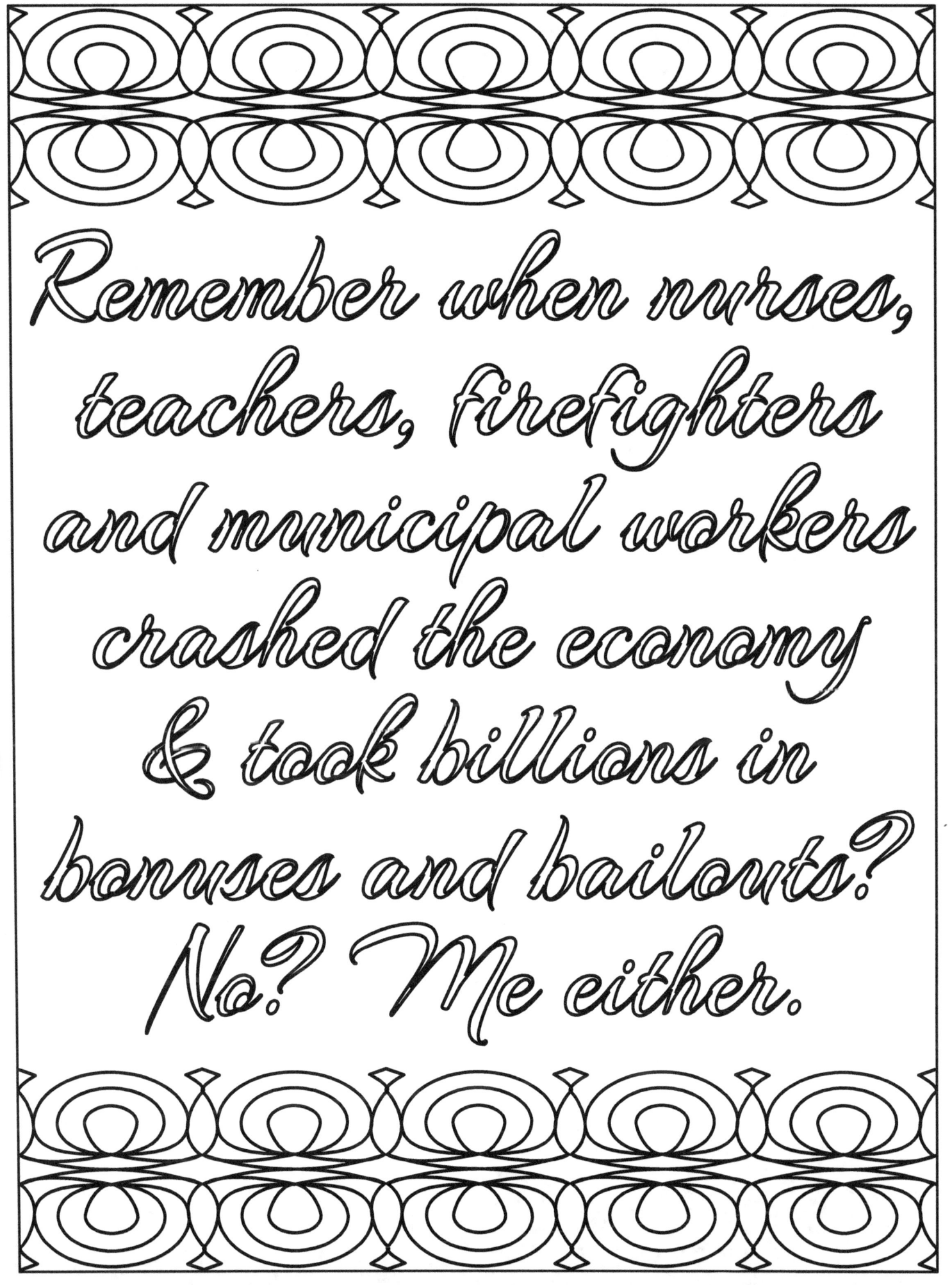

Remember when nurses, teachers, firefighters and municipal workers crashed the economy & took billions in bonuses and bailouts? No? Me either.